Competency Management for the Emergency Department

Contributing Authors:

Adrianne E. Avillion, DEd, RN
Barbara A. Brunt, MA, MN(c), RN, BC
Gwen A. Valois, MS, RN, BC
Jane G. Alberico, MS, RN, CEN

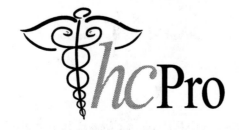

Competency Management for the Emergency Department is published by HCPro, Inc.

Copyright 2005 HCPro, Inc.

All rights reserved. Printed in the United States of America.   5   4   3   2   1

ISBN 1-57839-688-3

No part of this publication may be reproduced, in any form or by any means, without prior written consent of HCPro or the Copyright Clearance Center (978/750-8400). Please notify us immediately if you have received an unauthorized copy.

HCPro, Inc., is not affiliated in any way with the Joint Commission on Accreditation of Healthcare Organizations, which owns the JCAHO trademark.

Adrianne E. Avillion, DEd, RN, Contributing Author
Barbara A. Brunt, MA, MN(c), RN, BC, Contributing Author
Gwen A. Valois, MS, RN, BC, Contributing Author
Jane G. Alberico, MS, RN, CEN, Contributing Author
Melanie Roberts, Managing Editor
Lauren Rubenzahl, Copy Editor
Mike Mirabello, Senior Graphic Artist
Patrick Campagnone, Cover Designer
Jean St. Pierre, Director of Operations
Emily Sheahan, Group Publisher
Suzanne Perney, Publisher

Advice given is general. Readers should consult professional counsel for specific legal, ethical, or clinical questions.

Arrangements can be made for quantity discounts.

For more information, contact:
HCPro, Inc.
200 Hoods Lane
P.O. Box 1168
Marblehead, MA 01945
Telephone: 800/650-6787 or 781/639-1872
Fax: 781/639-2982
E-mail: *customerservice@hcpro.com*

Visit HCPro at its World Wide Web sites: *www.hcpro.com* and *www.hcmarketplace.com*

Contents

List of figures vi

About the authors vii

Preface ix

How to use this book xiii

Chapter 1: Why is competency validation required? 1

    Regulating competence 3
        Protecting the public 3
    JCAHO 6
        Standard HR.1.20 7
        Standard HR.2.10 7
        Standard HR.2.20 9
        Standard HR.2.30 10
        Standard HR.3.10 11
    Competency and litigation 11
    Case study: Surveyors tracing for competent care 12
    References 14

Chapter 2: What is competency validation? 15

    Competency-based education 17
    Defining competencies 23
    Classifying competencies by level and domains 23
        Domains of competency 23
        Levels of competency 24
    Who performs competency validation? 25
    Mandatory training v. competencies 26
    Mapping competencies for orientation, annual assessments .27
    Methods to validate competencies 29
        Posttests 29
        Observations of daily work 30

Case studies 30
Peer review/360° evaluation 30
Exemplars 30
Simulated events 31
Quality-improvement monitors 31
Scheduling and organizing the competencies 31
References 32

Chapter 3: Include competency validation in job descriptions and the performance-evaluation process 33

The benefits 36
JCAHO expectations 36
Key elements of a competency-based job description 38
    What makes a job description competency- or performance-based? 38
    Essential and nonessential functions 39
    Organizational competencies 41
    Rating scale and definitions 41
    Performance narratives 42
Compliance tips for HR.3.20 43

Chapter 4: Training staff to perform competency validation 45

Developing a competency assessment training program 47
    Purpose 48
    Principles of adult learning 48
    Learning styles 49
    Maintaining objectivity 49
    Offering constructive criticism 50
    How to assess competency consistently 50
Identifying your competency assessors 51
Peer review 55
Keeping your validation system consistent 56
Incorporating age-specific competencies 58
Documentation and recordkeeping 63
Conclusion 64
References 64

Chapter 5: Keep up with new competencies 65

    Potential categories for new competencies 67
        New equipment 67
        Interpersonal communications 68
        New patient populations 69
        New treatment measures 69
        New medications 70
        Research endeavors 70
    Guidelines for new competency development 70
    Best practices for the implementation of new competencies 75
        Competency skills fairs 75
        Drills and simulations 76
        Performance improvement monitors 77
        Return demonstration/observation 77
        Self-assessment 78
    Dimensions of competencies 79
    References 80

Chapter 6: Using your skills checklists 81

    Difference between orientation checklists and skill checklists 85
        Developing orientation checklists 86
    Skills checklists for annual competency assessment 99
        Determining what skills to evaluate 99
        Developing the skills checklists 99
        Identifying who can complete the checklists 99
        Keeping track of who has been evaluated 100
            The Competencies Analyzer 100
        Determining what happens when staff cannot perform competencies ... 102
        Other methods to validate competence 102
    References 105

How to use the files on your CD-ROM 107

ED—Emergency Department 111

ALL (General, All Units) 143

List of figures

Figure 2.1: Comparison of CBE and traditional education 18
Figure 2.2: Sample competency-based program policy 19
Figure 3.1: Essential functions 40
Figure 3.2: Rating scale and definitions 42
Figure 3.3: Compliance tips for HR.3.20 43
Figure 4.1: Successful completion of competency assessment training form 54
Figure 4.2: Patient populations and age ranges 59
Figure 4.3: Age-specific competency assessment form 61
Figure 5.1: New competency assessment checklist 73
Figure 6.1: Skills checklist template 84
Figure 6.2: Competency-based orientation checklist 87
Figure 6.3: Nursing assistant orientation checklist 93
Figure 6.4: Competencies tracking sheet 101

About the authors

Adrianne E. Avillion, DEd, RN

Adrianne E. Avillion, DEd, RN, is the president and owner of AEA Consulting in York, PA. She specializes in designing continuing education programs for healthcare professionals and freelance medical writing. Avillion also offers consulting services in work redesign, quality improvement, and staff development.

She has published extensively and has served as editor of the first and second editions of *Core Curriculum for Staff Development*, published by the National Nursing Staff Development Organization (NNSDO). She also is a frequent presenter at conferences and conventions devoted to the specialty of continuing education and staff development. Avillion is the vice president of the board of directors of NNSDO and holds a master's degree in nursing and a doctorate in adult education from Penn State University.

Barbara A. Brunt, MA, MN(c), RN, BC

Barbara A. Brunt, MA, MN(c), RN, BC, is manager of nursing education and staff development for Summa Health System in Akron, OH. She has held a variety of staff development positions, including educator, coordinator, and director for the past 26 years. Brunt has presented about a variety of topics both locally and nationally and has published numerous articles and chapters in books. She served as a section editor for the first and second editions of *The Core Curriculum for Staff Development* and was part of the task force that revised the *Scope and Standards of Practice for Nursing Professional Development*.

Brunt holds a master's degree in community health education from Kent State University and is currently finishing a master's in nursing from the University of Dundee in Scotland. Her research has focused on competencies. Brunt maintains certification in nursing professional development, as well as medical-surgical nursing. She has been active in numerous professional associations and has received awards for excellence in writing, nursing research, leadership, and staff development.

Gwen A. Valois, MS, RN, BC

Gwen A. Valois, MS, RN, BC, is the director of organizational development at Medical City Dallas Hospital in Dallas. She has clinical expertise in pediatrics and has served for more than 25 years in various clinical educational and leadership roles.

Valois received her BSN from Texas Woman's University, received her master's degree in human resource management and development from National Louis University, and holds certification from American Nurses Credentialing Center in nursing professional development.

Jane G. Alberico, MS, RN, CEN

Jane G. Alberico, MS, RN, CEN, has more than 30 years of nursing practice in healthcare. She received her bachelors of science from the University of Kentucky and master's degree in health science instruction, with a minor in healthcare administration from Texas Woman's University.

Alberico is a certified emergency nurse whose clinical expertise includes medical-surgical, home health, pain management, and emergency care. She has served in faculty and leadership roles in school and hospital settings. She is a national speaker for various topics and is currently the supervisor for clinical education at Medical City Dallas Hospital in Dallas.

Preface

Before you use any methodology for validating and assessing the competency of your nurses to deliver safe patient care, it is essential that you have a system in place for verifying that your nurses are who they say they are prior to allowing them on your unit.

That might sound obvious, but stories of nurses faking credentials, hopping from job to job in various states, and harming patients are stark reminders that you must be diligent in verifying any nursing applicant's licensure, criminal background, education, and employment history.

Unfortunately, the nurse-credentialing process in your facility may be like many others across the country: inadequate. Nurses who have had action taken against them by another state nursing board, have a criminal history, or have incomplete education may slip by and end up working in direct contact with your patients, making those patients vulnerable and your facility liable.

In fact, most facilities don't subject nurses to the kind of stringent credentialing process they apply to physicians. But considering how much closer to patients your nurses work, it might be in your—and your patients'—best interest to take another look at that discrepancy.

In Chapter one, we will discuss the Joint Commission on Accreditation of Healthcare Organization's (JCAHO) expectations for verifying your nurse applicants' qualifications, but those do little to clear up the deficiencies that surround this issue. Although your hospital may be compliant under JCAHO because it follows policies and regulations when hiring nurses, you should inspect your organization's policies to see whether they protect your patients and sufficiently screen applicants for dangerous nurses or imposters.

Credentialing nurses falls to the human resources (HR) department in most facilities, and the medical staff office handles physician and advance-practice registered nurse credentialing. For advice on credentialing nurses, HR administrators should consult their colleagues in the medical staff office, who most likely already have an established credentialing process in place.

Here are some steps you can take to verify nurses' credentials and to ensure your patients' safety and your facility's integrity:

Step 1: Gather applicant information

The application for employment should be thorough and should obtain the information needed to ensure patient safety in your facility. Ask for the following:

- The applicant's name and any other names he or she has used (e.g., a maiden name)

- Education, degree obtained, and name and location of education institution

- Professional licensure, state in which the license was issued, date issued, license number, and expiration date

- Disciplinary actions on the license

- Specialty certifications

- Employment history

Also determine whether the applicant has ever been convicted or pleaded guilty or no contest to any

- criminal charges (other than speeding violations)

- drug or alcohol-related offenses

If he or she has, ask him or her to specify the charges and the dates on which they occurred. Finally, inquire whether he or she has ever been suspended, sanctioned, or otherwise restricted from participating in any private, federal, or state health insurance program (e.g., Medicare or Medicaid) or similar federal, state, or health agency.

Step 2: Verify applicant's information

Verify the information you obtained on the application to the best of your ability. Even if you don't find anything, document each verification step to further reduce your hospital's liability.

Some facilities hire a third party to verify this information, but most often the HR department does it. Either way, make sure there's a specific, established process.

The best method of checking an applicant's qualifications is to use primary source verification, including education, licensure, and past employment. For the most accurate and up-to-date information, you should contact the boards by phone and check the state board in every state that the applicant nurse has worked. Most state licensing boards post licensure information on their Web sites.

Consider running criminal background checks on all your applicants, even if your state nursing board runs checks of its own—nurses may have committed a crime after receiving their licenses. In most states, the responsibility is on nurses to notify the state board if they are convicted of a crime, but they may or may not do so, which puts your facility at risk.

Another important part of the process is to check federal sanctions lists. If you hire a nurse who has been sanctioned by the Office of Inspector General or General Services Administration, you could be fined thousands of dollars. Reasons for sanctions include everything from defaulting on student loans to Medicare fraud.

Here are some other potential "red flags" to consider:

- **Gaps in job history:** HR professionals are well aware of this red flag, but be sure to ask about the gaps. Understand that there could be a perfectly good explanation for it such as the birth of a child or a family emergency.

- **Moving from state to state:** When applicants move around a lot, their licensure information could be buried or lost. Therefore, be sure to check the status of the license in each state in which they practiced.

- **Job hopping:** HR professionals are well aware of this pattern as well, and they will look twice at any applicant with evidence of it. But be sure to call each employer and verify that there were no disciplinary actions taken against the nurse.

Step 3: Continually verify employee's license after hire date

Most facilities check nurses' licenses when they are up for renewal to make sure that they are current and active. However, it is crucial that you institute a process to check licenses more often as well.

Ensure that your policy spells out that it is the nurse's responsibility to report any disciplinary action taken against his or her license over the course of the year. If your nurses do not report such action, they could be working on your unit with a suspended or inactive license and you would have no idea.

Creating a new credential-verification process or updating your current process may sound like an overwhelming task. It is, however, one too important to ignore.

How to use this book

Competency Management for the Emergency Department will help you understand the basics of competency validation and assessment and discuss the steps you need to take to develop a process for performing these assessments at your organization.

In addition, this book provides you with sample tools that will help you get started.

The book contains 39 sample competency validation skill sheets. The first page of both the Emergency Department and General, All Units sections contain a table of contents, which lists the name and page number of each skill sheet.

All of the content in the skill sheets was contributed by Summa Health System Hospitals in Akron, OH, and South Shore Hospital in Weymouth, MA. This content has been reprinted with the permission of those organizations.

Customizable, electronic versions of all of the skill sheets can be found on the CD-ROM accompanying the book. Instructions on how to download these forms from your CD-ROM and on to your computer begin on p. 109.

We've also included a copy of the "Competencies Analyzer" on your CD-ROM. This easy-to-use Excel spreadsheet will help your unit or department managers organize their competency assessment program.

Putting your skill sheets to work

The template used to standardize the appearance of these skill sheets appears on your CD-ROM. Save this blank template to your computer and use it to create additional skill sheets for your organization.

Duplicate this blank sheet as many times as needed. Type in content as you would into any table created using Microsoft's word-processing software to customize the sheets to fit your organization's needs using the information discussed in this manual.

HOW TO USE THIS BOOK

Name: _____ Date: _____

Skill: [_____]

Steps	Completed	Comments

Self-assessment	Evaluation/validation methods	Levels	Type of validation	Comments
☐ Experienced ☐ Need practice ☐ Never done ☐ Not applicable (based on scope of practice)	☐ Verbal ☐ Demonstration/observation ☐ Practical exercise ☐ Interactive class	☐ Beginner ☐ Intermediate ☐ Expert	☐ Orientation ☐ Annual ☐ Other _____	

_____   _____
Employee signature   **Observer signature**

Here is a quick look at one of the skill sheets:

Name, Date, Skill—This section includes a space for the name of the employee whose competency is being validated, the date the validation is taking place, and the name of the skill being validated. Consider adding a second employee identifier, such as the nurse's license number, to this section.

We have already provided the name of the skill for each of the skill sheets included in the manual. As we discuss in Chapter 2, however, all the competencies validated by your organization will not be technical or skill-based competencies, such as using a blood-glucose meter. Therefore, when customizing these sheets for validation of an interpersonal competency or a cultural competency, consider changing the term "skill" to "behavior" as a more accurate way to incorporate the elements required of these competencies.

Steps, completed, comments—This section is set up in a typical checklist format. After each step is successfully completed, the validator would add a check to the "Completed" column. Consider changing the term "steps" to "performance criteria" when creating sheets for competencies that may not conform to a step-by-step format. The validator can use the "Comments" column to record statements such as "needs reinforcement for steps" or "reteaching required."

Self-assessment—The validator should ask the employee to do a self-assessment of his or her competence on the skill being validated. Use this section to check off the appropriate response.

Evaluation/validation methods—This box contains some of the more common methodologies used to validate competencies. The validator should note which method was used in association with the skill sheet to validate the competency.

Levels—Consideration for the level of proficiency should be made when validating competencies (refer to Chapter 2). The level of proficiency (i.e., beginner, intermediate, expert) should coincide with the experience level of the employee. Should the level not coincide, then remediation should be planned to achieve the desired level of competence.

Type of validation—In this section, the validator can specify whether this competency validation tool was used during orientation, during an annual competency assessment, or at another point during the competency validation process.

Employee observer signatures—Have both the employee and the validator (i.e., observer) sign the completed tool. This helps ensure that the employee was an active participant in the process and that he or she understands and acknowledges this piece of the competency validation process.

Chapter 1

Why is competency validation required?

CHAPTER 1

Why is competency validation required?

Regulating competence

Does it seem like you are visited by regulatory survey teams every day? Sometimes the survey is announced and sometimes it's a surprise, but every time the surveyors—regardless of who they represent—are concerned about "competency."

The definition of this word is in the eye of the beholder. The *American Heritage Dictionary*, for instance, defines competent as "having sufficient ability; capable."[1] In healthcare, however, it's not so simple. Your healthcare staff make decisions and carry out responsibilities and job duties that affect patient's lives. When the goal is to achieve positive patient outcomes—whether to cure or manage a chronic disease process or to allow someone to die a dignified death—is "sufficient ability" going to be good enough? Should competency only apply to clinical bedside nursing? Should an RN case manager have to meet the same competency requirements as a critical-care staff nurse? No, no, and no.

Protecting the public

Regulatory agencies are rampant in the healthcare industry. Their purpose is to protect the public and to ensure a consistent standard of care for patients and families. Initially, there was only the Joint Commission on Accreditation of Hospitals (JCAH, which was renamed the Joint Commission on Accreditation of Healthcare Organizations, or JCAHO, in 1987). Ernest Codman, a physician, proposed the standardization process for hospitals in 1910. The American College of Surgeons (ACS) developed the Minimum Standards for Hospitals in 1917 and officially transferred its program to the JCAH in 1952. A trickling of new agencies followed, and in 1964, the JCAH started charging for surveys.[2] Now the list of regulators looks like alphabet soup. Political debates regarding the effectiveness of these agencies have multiplied in recent years. In July 2004, for example,

Chapter 1—Why is competency validation required?

the Centers for Medicare & Medicaid Services (CMS) began criticizing the validity of JCAHO accreditations. However, since its inception, the JCAHO has never had federal oversight.[3] In some cases, criteria for federally mandated CMS regulatory standards may exceed those of JCAHO.

For acute-care facilities, the agencies that "oversee" patient care and thus require competency assessment may now include (but are not limited to) the following:

- JCAHO
- CMS
- National Quality Foundation and the Leapfrog Group
- State departments of health and human services
- State medical foundations
- American Nurses Association (ANA)
- State Board of Nurse Examiners (BNE)
- Health Quality Improvement Initiatives
- Occupational Safety and Health Association (OSHA)
- College of American Pathology (CAP)
- Office of Inspector General
- Quality improvement organizations
- American Health Research and Quality
- The Food and Drug Administration
- Centers for Disease Control and Prevention (CDC)

Add to this a list of your hospital's competency assessment initiatives. Most of these initiatives revolve around the mission, vision, and value statements for the organization. Indicators may include

- patient satisfaction
- physician satisfaction
- employee health and pride
- fiscal responsibility
- community involvement
- risk management

Chapter 1—Why is competency validation required?

Those of us working in healthcare started our careers wanting to improve human life, and it is frustrating at times when it seems the bureaucracy of regulatory mandates keeps growing. But the business of healthcare must consist of personnel who are both caring and able to perform their job safely and correctly. Remember that the provision of quality care and services depends on knowledgeable, competent healthcare providers. Every organization should have a competency plan in place to ensure that performance expectations based on job-specific position descriptions are consistently met.

Your competency plan must be designed with consideration given to

- the mission, vision, and values of your organization
- the needs of patients and families served
- the extended community
- new services or technologies planned for future services
- special needs required for particular healthcare situations
- current standards of professional practice
- applicable legal and regulatory agency requirements
- hospital policies and procedures

In addition, the organization should also foster learning on a continual basis. The chief executive officer should mandate this learning environment and hold the leadership team and staff accountable for expected outcomes.[4] The entire organization must foster a work environment that helps employees discover what they need to learn for self-growth.

What's the return on this investment? A positive patient/family outcome. The outcome may be improved health, the ability to mange a chronic disorder, or even a dignified death.

A consistent process for competency assessment is essential throughout the organization for all job classes, contract personnel, and, when indicated, affiliating schools. There must be a centralized, organized approach that moves seamlessly throughout the continuum of care and ensures the same standard or practice for all of the patients and families it serves. If your main policies and procedures say one thing but certain departments or units develop their own policies and procedures that say something else, you are in trouble.

Chapter 1—Why is competency validation required?

Generating tons of paperwork does not ensure competency in practice. Use the KISS method: "Keep it simple, smarty." Although documenting that standards are being met is important, regulatory surveyors are moving away from looking at paper. The trend is to interview patients, staff, physicians, vendors, and members of the leadership team to see evidence of compliance. And now more than ever, there are expectations to move beyond merely verifying whether nurses are "competent." Thanks in part to advances in technology, nurses have been catapulted into more advanced and specialized care. Entire nursing divisions in hospital settings may now apply for Magnet recognition through the American Nursing Credentialing Center (ANCC). Designations like Magnet and the Malcolm Baldrige National Quality Award are raising the bar for practice by empowering nurses to demand excellence in delivering care.

In the future, instead of knowing the date a survey team will arrive at your hospital months in advance, the regulatory agency may show up at your door at anytime without advance notice. In fact, the JCAHO surveyors will begin doing so in 2006. Therefore, it is vital for you and your organization to be survey ready every day. Ongoing performance must be measured and assessed. If individual members of your healthcare organization do not meet the standards you've established, then the individual and the leadership team must develop a system in place for ongoing validation and assessment of personnel based on those standards. Remember: Competency assessment would be necessary even if it were not an accreditation standard.

It is worth framing this discussion around the expectations of regulatory agencies because understanding their motivations and complying with their recommendations will result in better understanding of what an effective competency assessment process should look like. What do these regulatory agencies want? In our discussion of the JCAHO below, we will also introduce the concepts of other state and federal agencies.

JCAHO

The JCAHO is still considered the leader in healthcare accreditation. Standards devoted to competency are woven through the JCAHO's accreditation manual, from the Leadership chapter to the Environment of Care chapter. It uses elements of performance (EP) to determine hospitals compliance with standards. The JCAHO's 2004 Human Resource (HR) standards listed below summarize its expectations for competency.[5]

Chapter 1—Why is competency validation required?

Standard HR.1.20

The hospital has a process to ensure that a person's qualifications are consistent with his or her job responsibilities.

This requirement pertains to staff, students, and volunteers who work in the same capacity as staff who provide care, treatment, and services. This includes contract staff.

It seems simple enough, doesn't it? Steve Doe applies to be an ED staff RN. HR department representatives compare what Steve Doe put on his application to the RN job description for an ED staff nurse to determine whether he meets the qualifications for the position. If the criteria on the job description states, "Licensed RN in the state of Texas. Minimum of two years recent clinical experience in an ED required. Current card in basic life support (BLS) for healthcare providers, advanced cardiac life support (ACLS) and pediatric advanced life support (PALS) required. Certified emergency nurse preferred," Steve Doe better meet the requirements.

As we indicated in the preface, the process for verifying these credentials is of utmost importance to the safety of your patients. Your organization needs a system to ensure that your nurses are who they say they are and have the experience and documentation to back it up. A surveyor may ask an ED nurse (who happens to be Steve Doe), "What is required to work in this department?" The nurse tells the surveyor what was required for his position. The surveyor may then ask for an ED staff RN job description and Steve's file to see whether the hospital did indeed verify that all the screening requirements were met and whether there is a record indicating that the requirements are still being met.

Standard HR.2.10

Orientation provides initial job training and information.

The EPs establish that this standard applies to each staff member, student, and volunteer at your facility. The EPs encompass the following:

1. The hospital's mission and goals

2. Organization- and relevant unit-, setting-, or program-specific (e.g., safety and infection control) policies and procedures

3. Specific job duties and responsibilities and unit-, setting-, or program-specific job duties related to safety and infection control

4. Cultural diversity and sensitivity

5. Patient rights and ethical aspects of care, treatment, and services and the process to address ethical issues

In addition, forensic staff (i.e., police who bring in prisoners) must know how to

- interact with patients
- respond to life safety codes
- communicate through appropriate channels
- define their roles in clinical seclusion and restraint

It is expected that, during orientation, the hospital assesses and documents the competency level of the new hire so by the end of orientation the person is deemed competent (sample orientation competency assessment tools for an RN and nurse assistant appear in Chapter 6). This standard highlights the fact that competence in nursing is not a one-size-fits-all arrangement. Although your ability to synthesize your competency assessment practices across your entire organization will ultimately determine your success, you must be able to customize your tools and process to their intended audience. However, keep in mind that the organization is not expected to shoulder this responsibility alone. Provision 5.2 under the ANA's Code of Ethics states that the nurse "is responsible to self as well as to others to maintain competence and to continue personal and professional growth."[6]

As a result, state BNEs' rules and regulations may dictate competency expectations. These regulations vary, but many discuss competency pertaining to

- role delineation for "respondant superiors" (i.e., adult nurse practitioners, licensed practical nurses, licensed vocational nurses, new grads, and unlicensed personnel)
- scopes of practice for patient care
- peer review
- informed consent
- medication administration
- pain management (including epidurals)
- conscious sedation/analgesia
- patient/family education
- blood administration
- growth and development v. age-specific care

Standard HR.2.20

Staff members, licensed independent practitioners, students, and volunteers can describe or demonstrate their roles and responsibilities based upon specific job duties relative to safety.

The EPs for this standard include

- risks within the hospital environment
- actions to eliminate, minimize, and report risks
- procedures to follow in the event of an adverse event
- reporting processes for common problems, failures, and user errors

This standard coincides with the introduction of the National Patient Safety Goals (NPSG) and new requirements by the JCAHO in 2004. The NPSGs are derived from a sentinel event advisory group, and the requirements are generally more prescriptive than other JCAHO requirements. They are based upon aggregate data following national trends of sentinel patient events. As of January 1, 2005, the JCAHO will incorporate NPSGs to the accreditation survey.[7] The NPSGs highlight the link between competent patient care and safety. To fulfill your hospital's mission of delivering safe patient care, there is significant value in validating healthcare professionals' competencies associated with these goals.

Also note that licensed independent practitioners (LIP) have been included in HR 2.20. An LIP is someone who is authorized by law and the hospital to "provide care and services without direction or supervision, within the scope of the individual's license and consistent with individually granted clinical privileges."[8] LIPs give medical orders for patient care. The individual is credentialed through the hospital medical staff committee.

Standard HR.2.30

Ongoing education, including inservices, training, and other activities, maintains and improves competence.

With this standard, the JCAHO expects that measuring competency at your organization is an ongoing process. In other words, it isn't enough for you to assume that your system for validating competencies at orientation will cover your employees for the length of their employment. EPs for this standard expect

- training when job responsibilities and duties change (e.g., when an ED nurse transfers to neonatal intensive care unit [NICU] but has never worked in an NICU setting).

- that participation in ongoing training will increase staff, student, or volunteer knowledge of work-related issues.

- ongoing education to be appropriate to patient needs, safety, and infection prevention and control and to comply with law and regulations. Staff must know how to manage and report unanticipated events.

- learning needs to be identified. Education is planned, implemented, and evaluated for effectiveness.

- documentation of learning for regulatory and legal requirements.

Most state boards of nursing mandate continuing education requirements for nurses who apply for relicensure. Hospitals striving for Magnet recognition through the ANCC are required to foster an environment of continual learning for nursing staff or risk losing their designation. This standard underlines the need for ongoing education and competency validation at your organization.

Standard HR.3.10
Competence to perform job responsibilities is assessed, demonstrated, and maintained.

Once again, this standard stresses that competency assessment be an ongoing process. An EP for this standard may be point-of-care testing for the CAP. For example, for CAP accreditation to be maintained, staff must be competent to perform point-of-care testing (POCT).[9] This testing goes beyond knowing how to do a fingerstick test for blood-glucose testing. CAP wants to know who is allowed to do POCT. Are staff involved in quality control testing and documentation as defined by hospital policy? What tests are allowed to be done outside of the main hospital laboratory, and what areas are allowed to do what? Examples of POCT that may need to be validated include (but may not be limited to)

- hemacult
- urine dipstick
- nitrazine pH
- blood glucose

Competency and litigation

Regulatory agencies and legal issues are conjoined in HR.3.10. What is the link? Competency assessment is "systematic and allows for a measurable assessment of the person's ability to perform required activities."[10] The EPs do not say that you have to use a certain form or have a certain methodology, but you do have to use a systematic measurable process.

In addition, whoever assesses competency must be qualified to do so. The leadership team must know the qualifications of the staff caring for the patient population served and is accountable and responsible for maintaining competent staff. For example, an ED nurse cannot deem another ED nurse competent in managing an overdose patient if the "assessor" has only managed one overdose patient. Peer review is critical to competency assessment, but careful consideration must be given to the process.

Plaintiffs' attorneys in legal cases use expert witnesses to verify issues related to competency. For example, the expert ED nurse called on the case of an overdose patient may manage several overdoses every day. The standard for excellence and competency in practice is likely embodied by this credible witness. If the patient had a negative outcome following a gastric lavage, the expert may be able to dispute the defendant organizations' method used to measure competency of ED staff nurses caring for overdose patients.

Case study: Surveyors tracing for competent care

The staff at Healthcare Hospital are in their second day of a four-day Joint Commission on Accreditation of Healthcare Organizations' (JCAHO) survey. Wanda, the nurse surveyor, is in the critical-care unit (CCU) focusing on a tracer patient named Mrs. D., who was admitted from the ED. Mrs. D. tried to commit suicide in the ED. She was lavaged for her overdose, intubated, and transferred to the CCU.

The JCAHO's tracer methodology strives to ensure that the same standard of care is used throughout the facility by retracing the care delivered to sample patients (or tracers), so Wanda asks the nurse manager to gather three caregivers associated with this patient's case. She also requests that she pull their personnel files because Wanda wants to first ask these nurses various questions regarding the care the patient received and their competency to deliver it. Then she'll verify whether accreditation standards have been met by reviewing their files. The three employees are

- a new graduate who is going through a critical-care internship

- a registered nurse (RN) with 25 years' experience in critical care

- a certified nursing assistant (CNA) who is a foreign nurse preparing to sit for the boards in the United States

Wanda also wants to review the nurse manager's file to verify that the manager meets the competency standards required of her as a member of the leadership team at this facility; she wants to know what training she has had to become a leader. Wanda then proceeds to walk around the unit and delves further into the standards for hospital accreditation.

Based upon federal and state regulatory requirements discussed in this chapter, can you think some of the important questions Wanda will ask the staff, physician, patient (if this vented patient could participate), and family?

Wanda may ask whether the new graduate is competent to take care of a ventilator patient. If so, how was that validated? If he or she is not competent, what is the action plan? If the nurse with 25 years' experience is her preceptor, how was she deemed competent? Can the CNA, who is a nurse in her country of origin, interpret the monitor strips correctly?

How would Wanda ensure the timely and accurate assessment of competencies for these personnel? Could she pull job descriptions? Performance evaluations? Competency checklists, or skillsheets? Is your organization ready for that?

Your organization must ask itself, "Are the right people taking care of the right patients for the right reasons?" Consider the following:

The decline of standards

A big city school system requires a student in the seventh grade to be able to read as well as a fifth grader, who must be able to read as well as a fourth grader, who, in turn, must be able to read as well as a third grader. What's wrong with demanding that a seventh grader be required to read like a seventh grader? How would you like to be operated on by a brain surgeon who graduated from a school that allowed its students to be a year and a half behind in their skills?

—*Author unknown*

References

1. American Heritage Dictionary, Third Edition, 1996.

2. JCAHO, "A Journey Through the History of Joint Commission," *www.jcaho.org/about+us/history/* (10/15/2004).

3. Tom Knight, "JCAHO Certification-Dissecting an Institution," *The Nurse's Lounge* (September 2004), p. 26.

4. Joint Commission Resources, *Assessing Hospital Staff Competence*, JCAHO (2002), p. 17.

5. JCAHO, *Comprehensive Accreditation Manual for Hospitals: The Official Handbook Refreshed Core*, (2004) pp. 210–220.

6. ANA, *Code of Ethics for Nurses with Interpretive Statements* (2001).

7. JCAHO, "Facts about the 2005 National Patient Safety Goals," *www.jcaho.org* (10/15/2004).

8. Joint Commission Resources, *Assessing Hospital Staff Competence*, JCAHO (2002), p. 8.

9. CAP Web site, *www.cap.org* (10/05/2004).

10. JCAHO, *Comprehensive Accreditation Manual for Hospitals: The Official Handbook Refreshed Core* (2004), pp. 210–220.

Chapter 2

What is competency validation?

Chapter 2

What is competency validation?

Competency is an issue that affects nursing personnel in all practice settings. Increased pressure from multiple healthcare regulatory agencies and the public necessitates comprehensive evaluation of staff competency. The public demands that nurses demonstrate their competence. This chapter provides information on competency-based education (CBE), as well as on levels and domains of competency. Responsibility for competency validation and the difference between mandatory training and competencies are outlined. The chapter describes methods to validate competence and options for mapping out or scheduling competencies.

Competency-based education

CBE is one approach commonly used to assess and validate competency. In many ways, CBE reflects a pragmatic concern for doing, not just knowing how to do. Competency models began to evolve during the 1960s as an approach to teacher education, and today CBE models are a widely applied approach to validating competence. In CBE, the learners' self-direction allows educators to act as facilitators to promote learners' goals and is compatible with adults' developmental needs.

JoAnn Griff Alspach, a well-known staff development expert, defined CBE as "an educational system that emphasizes a learner's ability to demonstrate the proficiencies that are of central importance to a given task, activity, or career." With this approach, the emphasis is on performance. Most CBE programs focus on outcomes rather than processes.

Common characteristics of CBE include a learner-centered philosophy, real-life orientation, flexibility, clearly articulated standards, a focus on outcomes, and criterion-referenced evaluation methods. Generally, CBE programs focus on a specific role and setting and use criteria developed by expert practitioners. CBE emphasizes outcomes in terms of what individuals must know and be able to do and allows flexible pathways for achieving those outcomes. A comparison of CBE and traditional education is provided in Figure 2.1.

Figure 2.1 Comparison of CBE and traditional education

Characteristic	CBE programs (Learner-centered)	Traditional education (Teacher-centered)
Basis of instruction	Student outcomes (competencies)	Specific information to be covered
Pace of instruction	Learner sets own pace in meeting objectives	All proceed at pace determined by instructor
How proceed from task to task	Master one task before moving to another	Fixed amount of time on each module
Focus of instruction	Specific tasks included in role	Information that may or may not be part of role
Method of evaluation	Evaluated according to predetermined standards	Relate achievement of learner to other learners

There are many benefits of a competency-based approach. These include

- having clear guidelines for everyone involved in the process
- encouraging teamwork
- enhancing skills and knowledge
- increasing staff retention
- reducing staff anxiety
- improving nursing performance
- ensuring compliance with the Joint Commission on Accreditation of Healthcare Organizations' (JCAHO) standard that all members of the staff are competent to fulfill their assigned responsibilities

A sample policy for a competency-based program appears in Figure 2.2.

Figure 2.2 — Sample competency-based program policy

SUMMA HEALTH SYSTEM HOSPITALS
AKRON CITY HOSPITAL
SAINT THOMAS HOSPITAL

POLICY: Competency-based program
SECTION: VI
PAGES: 4

Patient care services
Nonpatient care policy and procedure manual

SUBJECT:

Summa Health System Hospitals has adopted a competency-based program to ensure that nursing staff are prepared to deliver quality patient care. Assessment of competency begins with orientation and continues throughout employment. An evaluation of each nursing staff member's competency is conducted at defined intervals throughout the individual's association with the hospital. Performance appraisals may be used as a measure of ongoing competency of nursing employees. Nursing staff members have access to ongoing continuing education programs to enhance their competency.

DEFINITIONS:

Department of patient care services orientation: Consists of centralized orientation and unit orientation. Some areas also have a divisional orientation.

- **Centralized orientation:** Refers to the introduction, reinforcement, and demonstration of general required competencies that a nursing staff member needs to practice within any division of Summa Health System.

- **Divisional orientation:** Refers to the introduction and application of general practice concepts related to the division assigned. Divisional orientation is reserved for specialties such as critical care and operating room.

- **Unit orientation:** Refers to the clinical application of general and unit-specific competencies for a nursing staff member to practice on his or her assigned unit specialty or patient population. It also includes geographic and social orientation.

Figure 2.2 — Sample competency-based program policy (cont.)

Competency: Skill/activity identified by unit/division that must be successfully performed to promote quality patient care. Competency is concerned with what the individual can do in the provision of patient care.

- **Departmental competencies:** Competencies required for all staff assigned to direct patient care, such as Basic Life Support (BLS).

- **Divisional competencies:** Selected competencies required within a specific nursing division or specialty generally included in a curriculum specific to the division, or specialty, such as but not limited to

  Obstetrics
  – Neonatal resuscitation

  Critical care
  – ACLS
  – EKG interpretation

  Behavioral health
  – Nonviolent crisis intervention

- **Unit competencies:** Unit-specific competencies required for nursing staff members working on that unit/specialty patient population.

Competence assessment process

Competence assessment for nursing staff and volunteers who provide direct patient care is based on the following:

1. Populations served, including age ranges and specialties

2. Competencies required for role and provision of care

3. Competencies assessed during orientation

> **Figure 2.2** **Sample competency-based program policy (cont.)**

> 4. Unit-specific competencies that need to be assessed or reassessed on a yearly basis based on care modalities, age ranges, techniques, procedures, technology, equipment, skills needed, or changes in law and regulations
>
> 5. Appropriate assessment methods for the skill being assessed
>
> 6. Delineation of who is qualified to assess competence
>
> 7. Description of action taken when improvement activities lead to a determination that a staff member with performance problems is unable or unwilling to improve
>
> **Ongoing competence:** Refers to periodic assessment of selected competencies for the nursing staff member practicing within a division and on a specific nursing unit; may be centralized or division/unit specific.
>
> Required competency will include
>
> 1. annual performance appraisal
>
> 2. completion of mandatory organizational education and other inservices designated as mandatory for personnel
>
> 3. BLS healthcare provider course or renewal every two years (RNs, LPNs, technicians, medical assistants, emergency department nursing assistants)
>
> 4. BLS heartsaver course every two years (nursing assistants, unit secretaries)
>
> 5. unit competencies
>   Required specialty competencies will include the above as well as unit competencies. Each year unit-based competencies will be reviewed by the unit manager and required competencies changed based on individual needs of the unit, identified quality improvement needs or problems identified, changes in patient population, care modalities, technology, etc.

> **Figure 2.2** **Sample competency-based program policy (cont.)**
>
> A complete list of chosen unit-based competencies will be maintained in staff development.
>
> Staff not able to perform accurately any competency will be referred to the unit manager. They will be given 30 days to meet this competency and will not be assigned to a patient who requires that competency during that period. At the end of 30 days, if they cannot meet the required competency, they will be transferred from that area and reassigned to another area with an open position in which they meet the competencies. Continued failure to demonstrate required competencies leads to a practice plan for improvement and eventual termination.
>
> **Assessing competence**
>
> 1. Competency checklists will be used to assess demonstrated and ongoing competence. This ensures consistency in evaluating the steps to perform the skill.
>
> 2. When introducing new technology or procedures into the clinical area, the initial training is done by individuals with documented experience in that procedure (e.g., physician, nurses from that specialty, vendor representatives, etc.). A core group of staff members or a single individual is trained and confirms competency of other staff members after they personally demonstrate competence in that skill.
>
> 3. Ongoing competence will be assessed by an individual with documented competence in that skill. That competence may be determined by their role (e.g., advanced practice nurse, staff development instructor, unit manager, specialty coordinator, etc.), by their frequency performing the skill, or by already having demonstrated competence in that skill.
>
> _____
> Vice President, Patient Care Services
>
> _____
> Manager, Nursing Education and Staff Development
>
> *Source: Summa Health System Hospitals, Akron, OH. Reprinted with permission.*

Defining competencies

Confusion surrounding the competency movement is a result of the numerous definitions used to address this concept, and definitions vary widely. The definition used in this chapter is that competency is a broad statement describing an aspect of practice that must be developed and demonstrated, and competence is the achievement and integration of many competencies into practice, or the overall ability to perform. Competency is about what people can do. It is the integration of cognitive, affective, and psychomotor domains of practice. It involves both the ability to perform in a given context and the capacity to transfer knowledge and skills to new tasks and situations.

Classifying competencies by level and domains

Once an institution has a clear definition of competency, the next step is to classify competencies by level and domains.

Domains of competency

Dorothy del Bueno, a recognized expert in nursing competency-based education, described three domains of competence—technical, interpersonal, and critical thinking skills—which are often addressed in the literature about competence. Del Bueno developed a performance-based development system (PBDS) that focuses on these three aspects of practice.

The PBDS system provides initial assessment data about a nurse's ability to perform and identifies learning needs. Clinical judgment skills are assessed through a series of videotaped patient scenarios in which the nurse must identify the problem and outline what steps should be taken to solve that problem to assess his or her ability to recognize and manage patient problems and give rationale for interventions taken.

Patient Kardexes also provide the opportunity to assess the nurse's ability to prioritize scheduled activities for patients, and event cards are used to assess the ability to determine the priority for unscheduled events. If a task is a must-do event, the nurse must identify the appropriate action to be taken.

Audiotapes of various nurse-physician or nurse-nurse interactions assess the nurse's ability to recognize ineffective interpersonal strategies and identify interventions that could achieve more desirable outcomes. Some technical skills are demonstrated in a clinical laboratory setting, whereas others are demonstrated on the clinical unit. After the nurse completes the assessment, the assigned clinical instructor completes a profile documenting the assessment, develops an action plan that summarizes the findings, and identifies learning needs. The focus on technical skills, interpersonal skills, and critical thinking skills is helpful, although the initial evaluation of competence for new hires may be too time-intensive.

Some roles may require competencies in other domains appropriate for those roles. For instance, managers must demonstrate leadership competencies. In our increasingly diverse healthcare environment, it is important for staff members to demonstrate cultural competence when caring for patients of different backgrounds. Cultural competence is not only racial diversity, but also includes diversity in age, culture, religious beliefs, sexual orientation, and other demographic factors. Cultural competence builds first on an awareness of one's own cultural perspective and then acknowledges the perspectives of another culture on the same issue.

Levels of competency

Individuals function at various levels, and it is important to identify those differences in competencies. Pat Benner, a nurse theorist, differentiated five levels of skill acquisition in her novice-to-expert theory: novice, advanced beginner, competent, proficient, and expert. This book classifies competencies into three levels: beginner, intermediate, and expert.

Levels of performance are often differentiated by the ability to analyze and synthesize information. Beginners have limited exposure to the tasks expected of them and function at a basic level. With time and the development of expertise, they develop more skills and can identify potential problems and act accordingly—and they reach the intermediate level. Experts have a wealth of knowledge to draw upon and frequently anticipate problems and plan strategies to avoid them.

A competency on performing a respiratory assessment would be a beginning competency for a registered nurse (RN), whereas initiating actions to prevent or minimize complications based on one's assessment data would be an intermediate competency, and appropriately responding to subtle changes in respiratory assessment data would be a more expert competency.

Who performs competency validation?

After identifying expected competencies for each job classification, the next step is to determine who can validate competencies. This role will vary depending on the resources and types of personnel in the facility.

The American Nurses Association's *Nursing: Scope and Standards of Practice* addresses the mandate that nurses must provide care competently and keep up with current nursing practice. Individuals at all levels of the organization must assume personal responsibility to maintain their competence and ensure that they follow the system established by their organization to validate their competence.

Every organization has a responsibility to ensure that all staff members who provide patient care are educated appropriately and competent to fulfill their job responsibilities and meet acceptable standards. To meet the requirements of the JCAHO and other accrediting bodies, organizations must also ensure ongoing competence of employees. To do this, they must establish a competency system and determine who can validate competence.

Various individuals or groups with documented expertise in an area can validate competence of others. For instance, an agency could determine that either RNs or licensed practice nurses (LPN) can validate nursing assistants' competency in taking vital signs. For lifting and transfer techniques, someone from physical therapy or nurses could validate competency. For some skills, someone in one job category could validate the competence of another person in that same category. For instance, an experienced RN in critical care could validate the competence of a fellow RN in measuring cardiac output.

Organizations must identify clearly who can validate competencies and ensure that they have the appropriate education, experience, or expertise with that skill to perform the competency validation. Anyone who validates competence should be trained to do so (see Chapter 4) and should use an established competency checklist to ensure consistency with the evaluation process (see Chapter 6).

Mandatory training v. competencies

There is often confusion between competencies and mandatory training required by regulatory agencies or institutional policy. Most organizations require that all staff members review a variety of safety topics on a yearly basis, such as fire safety, dealing with emergency situations (e.g., cardiac arrests, disasters, hazardous materials, etc), and cultural diversity. Institutions have a variety of ways of achieving this task. Some distribute self-learning packets (SLP) containing the essential information and require everyone to review that material annually. Some SLPs may have a post-test, and some may require the individual to read the information. Institutions that have computer capabilities may require personnel to complete safety programs online. Some may hold face-to-face sessions which may or may not include some hands-on practice with the skill, for reviewing the information.

The difference between the mandatory training and competency validation is that the latter requires demonstration of the skill, whereas the former does not necessarily do so. To further clarify the difference, the list below outlines some of the common safety topics required by regulatory agencies:

- Cultural competence and ethical conduct
- Privacy and confidentiality issues (e.g., Health Insurance Portability and Accountability Act of 1996 [HIPAA] requirements)
- Fire safety
- Disaster preparedness
- Emergency codes
- Electrical safety
- Infection control and bloodborne pathogens
- Institutional safety plan and patient safety
- Back safety
- Emergency response to various threats (e.g., bombs, patient/family violence)

An example of competency is many organizations' requirement that personnel maintain competence in basic life support (BLS), which requires a staff member to complete appropriate courses as a healthcare provider, heartsaver, or advanced cardiac life-support provider.

The focus on competencies is on what the individual can do, not what they know, and competencies must be measured in a simulated or clinical setting. One example of a competency that can be demonstrated without specific patient contact is blood glucose testing. Any healthcare provider who tests blood sugar results must get an accurate reading because treatment is based on those results. The lab can provide a contrast material to the units so individuals can run a sample and send their results to lab. They can determine the accuracy of the individual's reading and ability to use the machine correctly by comparing their results with the test material.

Mapping competencies for orientation, annual assessments

There are a variety of ways to determine which skills should be evaluated each year. Selected competencies can be based on the needs of an individual unit, identified quality-improvement needs or problems, changes in patient population, care modalities, or new technologies. Summarized performance appraisal results could be used to indicate the particular competencies staff members need to develop further. Skills that are not used frequently but that present high risk to the patient can also be validated. Most institutions required some safety training annually, as well as BLS courses; these can also be part of the competency process. Many organizations are working toward integrating their performance appraisal and competency management systems. This is discussed further in Chapter 3.

Elizabeth Parsons and Mary Bona Capka suggest a model to determine how frequently skills should be assessed based on risk. Although this may be more detailed than necessary for some organizations, it may be helpful to identify high-risk procedures. The following are the key factors in their model:

- **Incident frequency.** This is determined by a rating scale that includes occurrence, quality improvement, and compliance data. Occurrence scores are ranked on a Likert-type scale (e.g., 5 = daily; 4 = once a week; 3 = once per month; 2 = once in six months; 1 = once per year or less; 0 = never). Incidents are defined as untoward incidents, equipment problems, staff noncompliance, or infection control data reported in the past 12 months. The more incidents, the higher the score.

- **Use/performance frequency.** This identifies the equipment use or competency performance. It uses the same Likert-type scale as the incident frequency scale with reversed scoring (e.g., 5 = once per year or less; 1 = daily). If procedures are performed infrequently, important steps may be inadvertently omitted. The more frequently the staff member performs the competency, the lower the score.

- **Patient/operator risk.** This scale scores each item according to the risk to the patient or operator if the competency is performed incorrectly. The highest score (i.e., 5 = operator or patient death) is assigned to competencies for which there is great risk to the patient or staff member, where the lowest score (i.e., 1 = barely any risk) is used if there is no significant risk to patient or staff member.

- **Skill complexity.** This score captures skills' complexity and is based on Benner's novice-to-expert model. Skills that the new graduate should be able to perform without supervision would rank lowest (1–2), whereas skills that require application of theoretical principles in creative and innovative ways score highest (9–10). In this manner, skills necessary to perform an identified competency factor into decisions made about the frequency of assessment.

The formula that Parsons and Capka used captured all these components, with risk being identified as the most crucial factor. Additional weight or value was given to the patient/operator risk score. Their formula is shown in the box below. Scores range from zero to 100.

Incident frequency (I) + user frequency (U) + skill complexity (C)
X patient/operator risk (R) = Total score (T), or
$$[I + F + C] R = T$$

For example, a skill such as providing immediate support for a cardiac arrest (e.g., BLS or advanced life support) would have a relatively high risk score. The incident frequency would encompass the number of untoward events during codes in the past year (1). User frequency would vary, but for most noncritical-care areas, it would be rated high (5) because it is not routinely performed in those areas. Complexity would be rather high (8) because a code is a complex patient care situation, and the risk would be high (5) because inappropriate performance of the competency could lead to patient death. A potential score of score of 70 could be obtained using the formula given above: (1 + 5 + 8) 5 = 70.

Your method for mapping competencies to be validated needs to be flexible enough to allow for changes or modifications based on environmental factors. For instance, a new piece of equipment might require staff to demonstrate competency in using that equipment. The system would need to be flexible enough to include that as an additional competency in a timely manner for the affected staff members.

Methods to validate competencies

It is important to realize that there are numerous ways to validate competencies. One of the most common methods is the skills checklist, which is described in Chapter 6. However, there are many other ways that competence can be validated.

Posttests

Posttests are one method to document cognitive knowledge and are sometimes used as a method to document competence. However, when competency is defined as the overall ability to perform, many tests do not have a performance aspect. One way that tests can be used is to document basic knowledge so participants don't have to take a course or program when they can show that they have the basic knowledge required in that course. For instance, someone with critical care experience could take a posttest to document that he or she has sufficient knowledge about a particular skill (e.g., cardiac monitoring) and, as a result, does not have to take that session of the curriculum. However, this would not take the place of validating his or her skills in the clinical area. Some tests may provide a written description, a videotape or audiotape, a live simulation, or printed or projected still pictures, and then present specific questions to which the test taker must respond. Del Bueno's PBDS system uses this approach to validate competency.

Observations of daily work

Observations of daily work, such as patient rounds or medical-record reviews, can be a means of validating competency. Specific interactions or skills can be directly observed as someone performs his or her work, and patient outcomes/documentation can be observed. This provides an opportunity for multiple observations and addresses one of the problems with checklists, which usually gather data from only one observation of a task. When staff know they are being observed, they have a tendency to go through all the steps correctly when they might not normally do so.

Case studies

Case studies are another means of validating competency. Individuals can describe how they would provide care for a particular patient or how they would deal with a particular scenario presented to them. These can also be used to address age-specific competencies. After someone describes how he or she would take care of a 37-year-old diabetic patient, the assessor could ask that person what he or she would do differently if the patient was 65 years old. Their description of the factors they would consider and how they would alter their care could be used to document their ability to care for patients of different ages.

Peer review/360° evaluation

Peer review, or a technique called "360° evaluation," is another method of validating competency. The 360° evaluation incorporates feedback from as many people who interact with a staff member as is feasible. For an RN, these people might include peers, LPNs, nursing assistants, representatives of other disciplines, and his or her manager. The use of different sources of information and different measures to evaluate competence increases validity.

Exemplars

Exemplars are narrative descriptions of practice. Individuals describe how they handled a particular situation, in essence writing or telling a story about it. Their narrative allows the clinician to describe the step-by-step progression of the incident, as well as the feelings, thoughts, and conclusions from their reflection of the situation. These exemplars can be part of portfolios that can provide concrete examples of competence in a particular area.

Simulated events

Simulated events, such as mock codes, can also be used to validate competency. For example, the instructor can use a mannequin in a bed to describe scenarios and ask the participants to respond appropriately. This provides an opportunity for practice and demonstration of skills in a non-threatening environment. Another example is the use of volunteers as simulated patients for staff to perform assessments or demonstrate various noninvasive skills. There are also various simulators that provide a realistic environment for demonstration of skills, but these can be costly.

Quality-improvement monitors

Quality-improvement monitors, if they reflect individual performance, are another method to validate competency. These are often related to quality-of-care issues such as falls, documentation, healthcare-acquired infections, and so on. With the ongoing emphasis on performance improvement and quality, most organizations have a quality-improvement program and quality monitors in place. For example, an institution may document compliance with the new HIPAA security requirements by having individuals without name tags approach staff members and tell them that they work for information technology services. They may ask the employees for their passwords to check the computer system or tell a secretary they are responding to a call about a computer problem and remove a piece of computer equipment from that secretary's manager's office. If the employee does not follow the established policy, feedback and follow-up is provided.

Scheduling and organizing the competencies

Once the competencies to be validated are determined, then the organization needs to communicate them to all staff members and provide the tools necessary to validate those skills. This can be done in a variety of ways. Access to the various checklists or methods to validate competencies should be available for all staff members to use during the validation process.

Some organizations may choose to have competency notebooks on each unit that include a tracking sheet of employees and a list of which competencies need validation for each level of personnel. Samples of skills checklists or other methods to validate competencies should also be included in the notebook. If there is a computer-tracking system in place, this can be used to map individual- or role-specific competencies. Then the person who performs the validation could enter that information directly into the computer system.

Some organizations may choose to put the responsibility upon individuals to make sure they are validated on the required competencies annually. In this case, the individual healthcare worker is responsible to have the appropriate person validate the skill and would be responsible to ensure that the appropriate documentation was completed. These data can then be used in the individual's performance appraisal.

Some institutions may schedule various competencies to be completed by everyone in a designated time frame (e.g., during the first quarter, two months before their annual performance appraisal). Others may allow competency validation to be done anytime during the year, as long as it is completed by a designated deadline date. Whatever system the organization uses to ensure that competence is validated must be communicated to all staff members, and a mechanism needs to be put in place to ensure that the process is followed.

A final step in the competency validation process is to set up a mechanism for ongoing review and evaluation of the process. Specific questions to be included in an evaluation of a competence assessment system are included in Chapter 6.

References

Alspach, JoAnn Griff. "Designing a competency-based orientation for critical care nurses." *Heart and Lung* 13, No. 6 (1984): 655–662.

American Nurses Association. *Nursing: Scope and standards of practice.* 3rd ed. Washington, DC: 2004.

Jeska, Susan D. "Competence assessment models and methods." In Karen J. Kelly-Thomas. *Clinical and Nursing Staff Development: Current Competence, Future Focus.* 2nd ed. Philadelphia: Lippincott-Raven, 1998: 121–144.

Joint Commission on Accreditation of Healthcare Organizations. *Comprehensive Accreditation Manual for Hospitals: The official handbook.* Oakbrook Terrace, IL: 2004.

Parsons, Elizabeth C., and Mary Bona Capka. "Building a successful risk-based competency assessment model." *AORN Journal.* 66, No.6 (1997): 1065–1071.

Chapter 3

Include competency validation in job descriptions and the performance-evaluation process

CHAPTER 3

Include competency validation in job descriptions and the performance-evaluation process

New technology, legislation, and accreditation standards are changing the job responsibilities of those employed at your organization almost every day. In some cases, these forces make it necessary for your organization to create entirely new job positions to keep pace and ensure safe, quality care. As a result, it is more difficult for hospitals to work with human resources (HR) to keep job descriptions current, create effective and realistic performance evaluations that are in sync with those job descriptions, and include these tools in a process for assessing initial and ongoing competencies.

We will provide further support for the underpinning theme throughout this book—manageability. That is, not only should you make your competency validation and assessment process compliant and effective, but it should also be manageable. This chapter discusses the elements required to build competency-based job descriptions. Competency-based (sometimes called performance-based) job descriptions state employee responsibilities in terms of practice standards, or how the responsibility must be demonstrated, rather than simply listing duties and responsibilities. Competency-based job descriptions, which can double as performance-evaluation tools, will also help you meet HR standards set by the Joint Commission on Accreditation of Healthcare Organizations (JCAHO).

Although these tools will take a good deal of time to develop, they will help your organization have a more streamlined system for developing performance criteria for your competency validation skill sheets, for assessing age/population-specific competencies, and for tying those assessments into timely performance evaluations. In this chapter, we will discuss

- the benefits of incorporating competency assessment into your job descriptions and performance evaluation tools

- what the JCAHO expects from hospitals in this area

- the key elements required of performance-based job descriptions

- practical tips for complying with JCAHO's challenging HR.3.20 standard, which expects timely completion of performance evaluations

The benefits

Your organization can expect several benefits from incorporating competency assessment into its job descriptions and performance evaluations, including the following:

- **Improved efficiency**—As long as you are willing to put the time and effort into building competency-based HR tools, your reward will be a more streamlined, JCAHO-compliant competency assessment process. The performance criteria in your job descriptions can serve as the foundation for your competency validation tools (e.g., skillsheets) and performance evaluations.

- **Improved patient safety**—Defining employees' job responsibilities by widely accepted standards or scopes of practice and holding employees to them will help your organization ensure that patient care is delivered in the safest way possible.

- **Improved employee satisfaction**—Employees need validation from their managers or supervisors about their job performance; They need to know what expectations they have or have not met. Well-developed HR tools composed of measurable performance criteria will make it easier for employees to receive this type of validation.

JCAHO expectations

According to the JCAHO, one of its competency assessment requirements, HR standard 3.10 (formerly HR5), ranks as the most-cited issue for JCAHO-accredited hospitals. HR.3.10 expects that hospitals assess staff competencies in relation to performance expectations outlined in their job descriptions.

CHAPTER 3—INCLUDE COMPETENCY VALIDATION IN JOB DESCRIPTIONS AND THE PERFORMANCE-EVALUATION PROCESS

If experience is any measure, it's no wonder organizations struggle with developing effective, time-tested competency assessment tools. In the past, a JCAHO survey team would visit a facility and make recommendations on how it could improve its competency assessment process or the tools associated with it. The facility would implement modifications based on those recommendations; then, three years later, a different survey team would come in and tell it something completely different. As a result, facilities had many different ideas about how to build an effective competency assessment program.

Scenarios like this one fostered the need for a process, mechanism, or tool to help hospitals develop strong competency assessment programs. A well-developed competency-based job description accomplishes this.

We discussed JCAHO's expectations for competency assessment in Chapter 1. As you may recall, JCAHO's HR.3.10 standard requires that your competency assessment process for staff, students, and volunteers who work in the same capacity as staff "providing care, treatment, and services" be based on, above all, populations served and the defined competencies required for each staff member. Therefore, there must be an effort to identify and validate age-specific or population-specific competencies (which we will discuss more in Chapter 4.) Do all healthcare professionals at your facility need to have these competencies validated? No—the JCAHO specifies that only staff who provide care, treatment, and services will need to have this done. Your housekeeping staff, for instance, do not need to have age-specific competencies validated.

However, keep in mind that there are clinical staff who aren't always licensed whose competencies will need to be validated. Pharmacy technicians, for example, are not licensed in many states, yet they fall into the category of clinical staff and deal a lot with medications. Although they're not licensed, pharmacy technicians clearly need to have an understanding of age-specific concerns regarding medication. Dietary aids are another example. They are unlicensed staff who do not assess or treat patients, but how they deliver food differs based on the age of patient. They may need to have age- or population-specific competencies validated.

The JCAHO also requires you to define a time frame for how often competency assessments are performed and (in HR.3.20) how often performance evaluations are performed. The JCAHO says this should be done at minimum once in the three-year accreditation cycle. Most important, however, is that you meet the objectives and goals associated with the time frame your organization chooses. If you fail to meet your expectations, the JCAHO will cite you.

This highlights the efficiency and effectiveness of a competency assessment process that incorporates both your job descriptions, which spell out the expectations, accountabilities, and competencies associated with the job, and performance evaluations, which allow managers to provide feedback on a regular basis and track employees progress toward those expectations, accountabilities, and competencies.

Key elements of a competency-based job description

What makes a job description competency- or performance-based?

The foundation for each employee's job description should be the position's qualifications, duties, and responsibilities. However, well-developed competency- or performance-based job descriptions at your facility must state employee responsibilities (i.e., essential functions and nonessential functions) in terms of expected practice standards—in other words, how the responsibilities must be demonstrated. Created by the department manager and understood by the HR department, these standards must have measurable, objective outcomes associated with them. The problem with many job descriptions is that they are written in a way that leads to subjective interpretations by supervisors.

Include an associated rating scale, which includes definitions that have been agreed upon across departments. This scale must be clear and easy to understand for everyone using it. Also include within job description an area for a supervisor to document how the employee met expectations in narrative format.

All the examples in the following section will be based on the job description of a float registered nurse, in the medical-surgical unit.

Essential and nonessential functions

Essential functions are those tasks, duties, and responsibilities that compose the context of the job (i.e., the means of accomplishing the job's purpose and objectives). The essential functions should be measurable statements that cover the major components of the job for which the person will be held accountable. An example of two essential functions and their expected performance criteria appear in Figure 3.1.

Functions listed as nonessential aren't unimportant—they just are not critical for the performance of the job position. They should be listed as specifically as possible and also should include performance criteria.

Figure 3.1 — Essential functions

1. Assesses and diagnoses patient and family needs to provide quality care to assigned patients.

- *Performs admission assessment within eight hours of admission or in accordance with specific unit standards.*
  - ❏ Consistently does not meet standards
  - ❏ Developmental/ Needs improvement
  - ❏ Consistently meets/ sometimes exceeds standards
  - ❏ Consistently exceeds standards

- *Identifies and documents nursing diagnosis on patients' plan of care within eight hours of admission.*
  - ❏ Consistently does not meet standards
  - ❏ Developmental/ Needs improvement
  - ❏ Consistently meets/ sometimes exceeds standards
  - ❏ Consistently exceeds standards

- *Identifies and documents patient/family/significant other of admission.*
  - ❏ Consistently does not meet standards
  - ❏ Developmental/ Needs improvement
  - ❏ Consistently meets/ sometimes exceeds standards
  - ❏ Consistently exceeds standards

Overall rating
- ❏ **Consistently does not meet standards**
- ❏ **Developmental/ Needs improvement**
- ❏ **Consistently meets/ sometimes exceeds standards**
- ❏ **Consistently exceeds standards**

Performance narrative

2. Develops, discusses, and communicates a realistic problem list (plan of care) for each patient, in collaboration with each patient/family/significant other in order to address all identified needs

- *Plan of care will include nursing diagnosis statement for each identified problem.*
  - ❏ Consistently does not meet standards
  - ❏ Developmental/ Needs improvement
  - ❏ Consistently meets/ sometimes exceeds standards
  - ❏ Consistently exceeds standards

- *Develops patient/family/significant other teaching and discharge plan as per unit standard*
  - ❏ Consistently does not meet standards
  - ❏ Developmental/ Needs improvement
  - ❏ Consistently meets/ sometimes exceeds standards
  - ❏ Consistently exceeds standards

Overall rating
- ❏ **Consistently does not meet standards**
- ❏ **Developmental/ Needs improvement**
- ❏ **Consistently meets/ sometimes exceeds standards**
- ❏ **Consistently exceeds standards**

Performance narrative

Chapter 3—Include competency validation in job descriptions and the performance-evaluation process

Organizational competencies

Job descriptions should also include organizational competencies—those that are expected across all departments of the organization for every employee. This will often require you to incorporate competency-based performance standards in sections devoted to (but not limited to)

- service
- teamwork
- communication
- respect for others
- time and priority management
- mandatory safety requirements
- leadership competencies

Rating scale and definitions

The rating scale portion of your job descriptions is extremely important. To develop a rating scale that is agreed upon across the organization, consider

- how many levels of ratings are required in order to differentiate performance

- how many standards can be identified, maintained, and discriminated in your performance appraisal process

- the reliability of raters across the organization in judging standards

- whether the rating scale produces improved performance and better communication

An example of a rating scale and definitions appears in Figure 3.2.

Figure 3.2 — Rating scale and definitions

Consistently exceeds standards	Performance consistently surpasses all established standards. Activities often contribute to improved or innovative work practices. This category is to be used for truly outstanding performance.
Consistently meets/ Sometimes exceeds standards	Performance meets all established standards and sometimes exceeds them. Activities contribute to increased unit/departmental results. Employees consistently complete the work that is required and at times go beyond expectations
Developmental/ Needs improvement	Performance meets most but not all established standards. Activities sometimes contribute to unit/department results. This category is to be used for employees who must demonstrate improvement or more consistent performance and/or for employees still learning their job.
Consistently does not meet standards	Performance is consistently below requirements/expectations. Immediate improvement is necessary.

Performance narratives

Performance narratives offer supervisors an opportunity to document their ongoing feedback and evaluation of staff performance. Your goal should be to establish consistency in rating performance across the organization. There is a lot of disagreement around what constitutes a good performance evaluation. However, the general thinking is that if you stick to criteria established in your job descriptions you will make it easier on employees and satisfy JCAHO surveyors.

To this end, a narrative box can be placed at the end of each essential function in your job description (see Figure 3.1). This differs from most traditional performance evaluations, which have space at the end of the form to document a narrative. This format would allow a supervisor to apply more specific feedback and recommendations.

CHAPTER 3—INCLUDE COMPETENCY VALIDATION IN JOB DESCRIPTIONS AND THE PERFORMANCE-EVALUATION PROCESS

> **Figure 3.3** — **Compliance tips for HR.3.20**
>
> Timely completion of performance evaluations is critical to the success of your entire organization and your JCAHO survey. To ensure that success, some organizations have established 30- to 90-day windows from the time the reviews are sent out to the time they are due for managers to get the work done. Here is some more advice from industry experts to reduce your turnaround time and reduce your risk of noncompliance with the JCAHO's HR.3.20:
>
> 1. **Keep your performance evaluations realistic.** A lot of organizations go to great lengths to design comprehensive performance evaluations that address every potential aspect of competency, but managers can't complete them because they are too complicated, says Bud Pate, REHS, practice director for clinical operations improvement for The Greeley Company, a division of HCPro, Inc., in Marblehead, MA.
>
> 2. **Post reminders.** The key to success is discipline, according to Glenn D. Krasker, MHSA, president of Critical Management Solutions, a consulting firm that specializes in medical error risk reduction in Wilmington, DE. It's best if evaluations are due on employee anniversary dates, rather than all of the organization's evaluations being due on the same date, so the workload is spread out over 12 months.
>
> 3. **Institute self-evaluations.** Help reduce the burden on supervisors by getting employees to complete a self-assessment of their job performance prior to the performance evaluation, which the manager will amend before it is sent to HR, says Katherine Chamberlain, CPHQ, a consultant in Gloucester, MA.
>
> 4. **Hold supervisors accountable.** Tie in supervisors evaluations and pay increases to the timelines of their completion of staff evaluations, suggests Krasker.
>
> 5. **Condense your evaluations.** Make sure your evaluations are not overly burdensome. Try to keep the document to one or two pages, says Pate.
>
> 6. **Automate the process.** Online performance evaluation tools help streamline the process because the forms are easily accessible to everyone and can be filled out quickly and legibly, says Deb Ankowicz, RN, BSN, CPHQ, director of risk management for the University of Wisconsin Hospitals & Clinics in Madison.
>
> 7. **Have a blitz day.** If managers are running behind schedule, reserve a conference room where they can work without interruptions to get their evaluations done, says Krasker.
>
> *Source: Adapted from* Briefings on JCAHO *newsletter, published by HCPro, Inc.*

Chapter 3—Include competency validation in job descriptions and the performance-evaluation process

The key to successfully incorporating your competency assessment process into the ongoing maintenance of job descriptions and the completion of performance evaluations is developing manageable tools. At the very least, these tools need to identify measurable performance criteria and promote consistent, agreed-upon methods for evaluating staff (based in part on the populations with which they work) and getting it all done in a timely manner.

Chapter 4

Train staff to perform competency validation

CHAPTER 4

Train staff to perform competency validation

Who performs competency validation within your organization? How are they trained to perform this important responsibility? Ideally, those who assess the competency of others are selected based on their clinical skills and ability to help colleagues enhance job performance. This means that they also possess tact and good teaching skills and receive appropriate training prior to evaluating colleagues' job performance. The opposite of this ideal situation is to have all staff assess the competency of others with little or no training, regardless of their teaching skills.

The truth is, most organizations fall somewhere between these two extremes. The purpose of this chapter is to help you design a practical training program for those staff members responsible for assessing the competency of others.

Developing a competency assessment training program

Who should be trained to perform competency assessment? First, understand that not all staff members should be trained to assess their colleagues' competency. Competency assessment is an acquired skill that not all healthcare professionals possess.

What qualifications should a competency assessor possess?

- Excellent performance of the competencies being evaluated
- Tact and the desire to help colleagues improve their job performance
- The desire to acquire/enhance adult education skills
- Demonstration of excellent interpersonal communication skills

Now that you know who should be trained, what should you include in the training program? The following components should be part of your competency assessment training and education program.

CHAPTER 4—TRAIN STAFF TO PERFORM COMPETENCY VALIDATION

Purpose

Learners need to understand the purpose and importance of a competency assessment program. You need to be able to demonstrate how job performance is enhanced and patient care improved by adhering to competency criteria. Use quality improvement and risk management data to prove your point. Learners must also understand that the Joint Commission on Accreditation of Healthcare Organizations (JCAHO) and other accrediting agencies expect staff members to demonstrate their competence, that such competence is evaluated on an ongoing basis, and that each staff member's competence is documented.

Principles of adult learning

Any education program that involves training adults to teach/coach other adults must include an overview of the principles of adult learning.

- **Adults must have a valid reason for learning.** Adults want proof that there is a need for learning (i.e., they want to know why it is important for them to participate in an educational activity). For example, suppose the ability to draw arterial blood gases (ABG) is a competency for all RNs on the medical intensive care unit. Some of them complain that this is a task performed frequently and they don't need someone observing them to validate their competency. If you are able to cite quality improvement data indicating a negative trend (e.g. infections, bruising, etc.) due to questionable technique, you can show them why there is a need for continual competency assessment. National data can also be cited to illustrate the need for keeping "on top" of a particular skill.

- **Adults are self-directed learners.** Adults direct their own learning. They want to feel that they have some control over what they learn and the manner in which they learn it. Adults also need to feel that their opinions matter and their learning needs are respected.

- **Adults bring a variety of life experiences to any learning situation.** Such life experiences can facilitate any learning activity. Even experiences not directly related to healthcare can enhance education.

- **Adults concentrate on acquiring knowledge and skills that help them improve their professional and/or personal lives.** Adults measure the importance of education by focusing on how new knowledge and skills will help them improve their professional performance or enhance their private lives.

- **Adults respond to both extrinsic and intrinsic motivators.** Adults must know how learning activities meet their extrinsic and intrinsic needs. Extrinsic motivators include things such as job promotions and raises in salaries. Examples of intrinsic motivators include enhanced self-esteem and an increase in job satisfaction.

Learning styles

When you assess competency, you are often in the position of teacher. Even though someone demonstrates competency, you may have suggestions to help improve some aspect of their skill. Include an overview of learning styles when you design your competency assessment training program.

- *Auditory learners.* Auditory learners assimilate knowledge by hearing. They prefer lectures, discussions, and audiotapes. They respond most favorably to verbal instructions.

- *Visual learners.* Visual learning is the most predominant adult learning style. Visual learners sit in the front of a classroom, take detailed notes, and respond to verbal discussions that contain large amounts of imagery.

- *Kinesthetic learners.* Kinesthetic learners learn best by "doing." They need direct hands-on involvement and physical activity as part of the learning experience.

Maintaining objectivity

It is important that those persons assessing competency maintain their objectivity. The training program should contain information about performing objective evaluations and not letting personal feelings—positive or negative—influence the outcome of the assessment.

Offering constructive criticism

This is one of the most challenging responsibilities of anyone who evaluates the job performance of others. The purpose of constructive criticism is to provide feedback on both strengths and weaknesses. Constructive criticism should motivate, reinforce learning, and identify the nature and extent of problems. One of the most important parts of constructive criticism is the development of a specific plan to help staff members improve their performance. Use the following four steps when giving feedback:

- **Step one: Identify the unacceptable actions**

  What is the staff member doing or failing to do that is not acceptable? Remember to focus on the employee's behavior, NOT on his or her personality. Give specific examples such as, "You broke sterile technique when you touched the IV tubing with your sterile-gloved hand;" not "You seem to be careless and not care if you endanger the patient by ignoring proper sterile technique."

- **Step two: Explain the outcome**

  What is it about the behavior that is unacceptable? How does it negatively impact productivity, patient outcomes, etc.? Be specific. Use descriptive terms instead of evaluative terms.

- **Step three: Establish the expectation**

  What is it the employee must do to correct unacceptable behavior? Again, be specific, and use objective, descriptive terms. You are describing actions to improve behavior, not evaluative comments about a person's personality.

- **Step four: Identify the consequences**

  What will happen if the employee corrects his or her behavior? What will happen if he or she does not?

How to assess competency consistently

One of the biggest challenges of any competency assessment program is the need for consistency among those persons doing the assessments. How do you make sure that one person is not too stringent and another too lenient? Are friends assessing friends' competency? Does this make a difference in the outcome? Are persons who dislike each other assessing each other's competency? Your training program must provide staff members with the tools and support needed to do proper competency assessment. This includes maintaining up-to-date policies and procedures, appropriate documentation checklists, and adequate education and training (a detailed description of these components is provided later in this chapter).

Consistency in documentation is as important as consistency in approach. The same tool template should be used by everyone. A procedure that describes how to document competency is needed.

Identifying your competency assessors

Can you identify competency assessors by title? Let's look at some common job titles that may carry with them the responsibility for competency assessment.

- **Preceptors:** The ability to perform competency assessment is an integral part of the preceptor role. The preceptor is necessary to the successful orientation of new employees. The essential qualities needed by competency assessors are also preceptor attributes. These qualities include the following:

    – Possesses excellent clinical skills, or, in non-clinical roles, excellence in job-specific skills
    – Demonstrates respect for colleagues
    – Acts as an excellent role model
    – Demonstrates outstanding interpersonal communication skills

    The assumption that preceptors adequately assess competency is based on the belief that your preceptor training program includes the essential components described earlier in this chapter. In order to increase the efficiency of training delivery, consider inviting staff members who need to be trained as competency assessors (but who are not preceptors) to the preceptor classes that offer training in competency assessment.

- **Nurse managers:** Nurse managers are generally not the best persons to assess clinical competency. In today's healthcare environment, nurse managers spend the majority of their time performing administrative duties such as staffing, budgeting, developing leadership, and handling performance issues. Their expertise in these areas, however, makes them able to validate such competencies in fellow nurse managers. Nurse managers rely on their staff members to possess clinical expertise, just as staff members rely on nurse managers for administrative expertise. Remember that in order to assess clinical competency properly, the evaluator must be able to demonstrate excellence in clinical skills. Nurse managers assess the managerial competency of their peers.

- **Staff development specialists:** Staff development specialists are the education experts within a healthcare organization. Their specific roles and areas of expertise determine whether they are involved in clinical competency assessment. For example, a staff development specialist based on the coronary-care unit who provides direct patient care as well as staff education is qualified to assess clinical competency. However, the staff development specialist who primarily offers management and leadership training and does not provide direct patient care is generally not qualified to assess clinical competency.

   Don't forget that staff development specialists must demonstrate competency in the adult education arena as well. Such competencies include program planning, teaching, and evaluating the effectiveness of education are essential to the persons specializing in staff development.

   Staff development specialists work with management and staff to design the organization's entire competency assessment program in addition to the program's training component. They provide the educational expertise that makes for a sound foundation for any competency program. But, like anyone else who is responsible for assessing competency, staff development specialists must be competent in the skills that they evaluate.

- **Staff nurses:** Staff nurses who demonstrate the necessary skills may also be part of a competency assessment program. It is important that they receive the necessary training. Depending on the arrangement of your clinical ladder or other similar programs, you may choose to have competency assessment as part of the requirements for promotion.

- **Nursing assistants:** Can you think of exceptionally competent nursing assistants in your organization? Training such nursing assistants to assess the competency of their peers is a definite possibility. As you develop a promotional ladder for nursing assistants, consider training those who are exceptional to participate in competency assessment.

- **Nonclinical staff:** Most healthcare organizations have competency assessment programs in place for nonclinical areas as well as for clinical areas. As your competency program develops and expands, don't forget to be on the lookout for nonclinical staff members who have what it takes to assess the competency of others.

You already know that you need to document competency achievement. Don't forget to document that your trainees have achieved competency in their ability to evaluate the performance of others. The following form is an example of a tool for such documentation.

Figure 4.1: Successful completion of competency assessment training form

Date: _____

Objectives: _____
_____
_____

Competency demonstration:
1. Explains purpose and importance of a competency assessment program
2. Incorporates the principles of adult learning as part of assessing competency
3. Recognizes various learning styles and meets the needs of learners representing these styles
4. Maintains objectivity when assessing competency
5. Offers feedback in a constructive manner
6. Is consistent in competency assessment approach
7. Documents results of competency assessment accurately and consistently

Trainer comments: _____
_____
_____

Learner comments: _____
_____
_____

Competency assessment training was successfully completed:

_____   _____
Trainer's signature and date   Learner's signature and date

Competency assessment training was not successfully completed:

_____
Trainer's signature and date

The following steps will be taken by the learner to successfully complete training:

Action	To be completed by the following date:
_____	_____
_____	_____
_____	_____

_____
Learner's signature and date

Peer review

The word "peer" is defined as a person or thing having the same rank, value, and/or ability—in other words, an equal. If an important part of your competency program is the concept of "peer review," be careful that you are truly asking peers to evaluate peers. For example, suppose City Hospital's competency policy/procedure states that competency is assessed via a peer-review competency-assessment program. City Hospital also has a career ladder for nurses that includes the following titles: staff nurse I, staff nurse II, and staff nurse III.

During a recent competency evaluation session, a staff nurse III (Carolyn) observes a staff nurse II (Amanda) performing the insertion of an intravenous needle. Carolyn documents that Amanda is not competent and needs remedial work. Amanda files a grievance with the hospital disciplinary board stating that Carolyn evaluated her unfairly. In part, the grievance read, "As a staff nurse III, Carolyn held Amanda to a higher standard, instead of evaluating her according to her experience at the staff nurse II level. Because City Hospital maintains that competency assessment is a form of peer review, Amanda was unfairly evaluated." The disciplinary board supported Amanda, and Carolyn's competency assessment documentation was removed from Amanda's file.

Sound far-fetched? Unfortunately, this kind of problem is not uncommon. Let's look at some pitfalls that might have contributed to City Hospital's (and Carolyn's) dilemma. Consider the following questions/comments:

- Did the policy/procedure clearly define the concept of peer review? Could this problem have been avoided by stating that competency is assessed by several types of staff members (i.e., peers and those functioning at a higher level according to the organization's career ladder)? If the policy is written in this manner, Carolyn could assess the competency of peers, subordinates, and those at a lower level than she on the clinical ladder as long as she is competent in the skill being assessed.

- Did Carolyn receive appropriate training in how to assess competency? Are the results of this training documented?

- Was it clear what had to be accomplished for competency to be achieved? Were the steps in writing and part of the competency assessment documentation tool? Did both nurses clearly understand what had to be demonstrated?

- Was objectivity maintained? Do interpersonal conflicts exist between Carolyn and Amanda?

Peer review is an excellent means of support and a worthwhile component of competency assessment. But be very careful that you define what you mean by a peer review. As in the case of City Hospital, if you fail to allow a more experienced nurse to evaluate a less experienced nurse or a subordinate, you may encounter serious problems. You may want to incorporate the definitions of various levels of expertise within your policies and procedures. Use the criteria established by your clinical ladder programs to delineate what levels of staff are able to evaluate other levels of staff. It may sound like a lot of extra work or being over-cautious, but this type of anticipatory planning prevents or reduces the number of grievances or union actions you encounter.

Keeping your validation system consistent

Nothing is as demoralizing as inconsistency in evaluation, and there are few things as challenging as ensuring consistency of approach among many different people. Here are some tips for helping to maintain inter-rater reliability among your competency assessors:

- Select your competency assessor based on the characteristics described earlier in this chapter. You may be tempted to have all members of the nursing staff assess the competency of others. In this day and age of nursing shortages and the need for complex nursing interventions, having everyone assess competency may seem like a quick fix to the problem of documenting competency assessment, but don't succumb to this temptation. In the long run, it will lead to disgruntled employees, failure to adequately assess competency, and a plethora of union and disciplinary grievances. Establish your criteria for selection, put it in writing in policies and procedures, and stick to it.

- The ability to assess the competency of fellow employees is in itself a competency. Successful completion of the training program on competency assessment must be documented. Failure to successfully complete the program demands that the trainee perform remedial work. He or she must not assess the competency of others until training is successfully completed.

- Avoid compromising objectivity whenever possible. If competency is assessed individually in an on-the-job environment, avoid pairing staff members who have known interpersonal conflicts. Likewise, avoid pairing staff members who are close friends. Either situation runs the risk of accusations of favoritism or prejudice. Consider having staff members from other units evaluate each other. Doing so may enhance objectivity.

- The steps that must be performed and how they are to be performed are clearly documented on the competency assessment form. Never assume that "everyone knows how to do this!" Failure to achieve competency can have dramatic consequences, including termination of employment. The only way to ensure consistency fairly is to provide a written guide delineating what constitutes successful competency demonstration.

- Develop a written checklist so that competency is evaluated on a step-by-step basis. The competency assessor must sign and date the checklist. The learner must also sign and date the checklist. Any remedial action plans must be documented along with targeted dates for achievement.

- The person assessing competency must document his or her evaluation findings. This task cannot be delegated to someone else. For example, suppose a busy manager asks one of her senior staff nurses to document a competency assessment for her. This is completely unacceptable. Competency assessment is just like any other type of nursing documentation: You do it, you document it.

- Have a plan in place to deal with persons who object to their competency rating. Include this plan in your policies and procedures. If a staff member is unfairly evaluated, he or she needs to know that there is a professional way to seek a reassessment. The steps that must be taken, including any necessary objective evidence, should be described in these policies and procedures.

- Policies and procedures must also describe the circumstances under which a grievance or other protest mechanism will be heard.

Incorporating age-specific competencies

The various physiological and psychological needs of each patient's age group is part of any well-designed competency program. The ability to implement age-appropriate interventions is critical to the quality and suitability of patient care.

The demonstration and corresponding documentation of age-specific staff competencies are important for a number of reasons. First and foremost, such competency validates the knowledge and skills of staff members. Appropriate knowledge and skill contributes to the quality of patient care and family services. And, finally, the JCAHO requires that age-specific (known as population-specific in the 2004 standards) competency be assessed on an ongoing basis and that the findings of these assessments are documented and maintained as part of the employee's file.

Age-specific competency requires proof of education and training, as well as the demonstration of skill achievement. During orientation, all employees must receive education and training concerning the specific patient age groups they will care for. Remember that this includes employees who, although not new to your organization, are new to a department or unit. For example, suppose that Martha has worked on an adult oncology unit for five years. She is transferring to a pediatric oncology unit this month. During Martha's orientation to pediatric oncology, the organization must provide her with education and training specific to pediatric oncology patients. This education and training must be documented and maintained in Martha's employee file.

Does age-specific competency mean that all care-givers must demonstrate competency of all age groups? No, this is not the case. Identify the age range of patients that staff members encounter most frequently in their work. Refer to the following table (Figure 4.2) for the age ranges of specific patient groups.

Figure 4.2 — Patient populations and age ranges

Patient population	Age range
Neonate	First four weeks of life
Infant	Up to one year old
Toddler	One to three years of age
Preschooler	Three to five years of age
School-aged	Six to 12 years of age
Adolescent	13 to 18 years of age
Young adult	19 to 44 years of age
Adult/Middle aged	45 to 65 years of age
Later adulthood/Geriatric	More than 65 years of age

A nurse who works on an adult oncology unit cares for patients in the young adult through geriatric age ranges. She or he must demonstrate competency in providing nursing care to patients who are young adults, middle-aged adults, and geriatric adults. Likewise, a nurse who works in a neonatal intensive care unit would need to demonstrate competency in providing care for neonates, not geriatric patients.

What are some efficient, cost-effective ways to achieve and demonstrate age-specific competencies? Let's start with education and training.

Simply attending an education program does not guarantee transfer of learning to the work setting. However, since healthcare science and research seems to bring new and exciting discoveries to the healthcare arena every day, part of the requirements of competency maintenance may involve participating in a specified number of age-specific education hours. These hours do not need to be offered exclusively in a classroom setting. Options such as self-learning packets, videos, or computer-based learning are cost-effective, efficient ways of delivering education and training. Successful achievement of educational post-tests measure learning or the acquisition of knowledge.

But, as we discussed earlier in this chapter, knowledge acquisition does not equate the ability to successfully transfer knowledge. How can we assess age-specific competencies? Ongoing competency may be evaluated in several ways, including direct observation, medical record review, and patient outcomes. Let's review the competency of Melanie, a nurse who works on an adult medical-surgical unit. What methodologies can we use to be sure that she is competent in providing care to geriatric patients?

- **Medical record review:** Are appropriate skin care nursing interventions documented? Is there documented evidence that safety measures are in place considering the patient's age and diagnosis? Has skin turgor been assessed? Identify specific interventions for the assessor to find within the medical record, including nursing care plans, nurse's notes, etc. You need to be specific to facilitate consistency of evaluation.

- **Direct observations:** Does Melanie provide care in a manner that incorporates age-specific concerns for the geriatric patient? In addition to observing Melanie as she actually provides care, you can assess patient outcomes and the environment. For instance, when assessing safety issues, determine whether the call-bell is within reach, whether non-skid slippers readily available, etc. Again, be specific about what exactly assessors need to evaluate. Select some universal geriatric issues and determine whether these issues are part of the patient's plan of care.

- **Equipment use:** Is equipment use adapted to the needs of the geriatric patient? For instance, if a geriatric patient is receiving intravenous hydration, are measures taken to avoid fluid overload, a potential danger for an elderly patient?

These are only a few of the ways to assess age-related competency. Remember that such assessment must be carried out consistently by all reviewers. This means that written guidelines must be established. The following template (Figure 4.3) is presented as a resource for the development of these types of criteria.

Figure 4.3 Age-specific competency assessment form

Date: _____

Objectives: _____
_____
_____

Mandatory attendance at ____ hours of continuing age-specific education completed. ☐ Yes ☐ No

Date of program   Title of program   Learner outcomes
_____
_____
_____

If education was not competed, the following corrective actions will be taken:

   Action   Target achievement date
_____
_____
_____

EVALUATION METHODS:

Medical record review:
_____
_____
_____

Direct observation of care:
_____
_____
_____

Observation of patient's environment:
_____
_____
_____

Figure 4.3 Age-specific competency assessment form (cont.)

Review of patient outcomes:

_____
_____
_____

Evaluator's comments:

_____
_____
_____

Age-specific competency was successfully demonstrated:

_____
Evaluator's signature and date

_____
Signature of nurse being evaluated and date

Age-specific competency was not demonstrated:

_____
Evaluator's signature and date

The following actions will be taken by the learner to achieve competency:

Action	Target achievement date
_____	_____
_____	_____
_____	_____

_____
Learner's signature and date

Documentation and recordkeeping

It is essential that your competency assessment program include appropriate documentation and maintenance of such documentation. Various sample checklists and templates are presented throughout this chapter. As a summary of important issues, let's review documentation components that are absolutely essential:

- **Assessment documentation must be dated.** Although you may think that this component is self-evident, it is astonishing how many times it is missed. The top of any form generally contains a space for the date, but all signatures should be dated as well. This decreases the chance of any discrepancies concerning assessment dates.

- **Identify the specific competency being assessed.** This includes the specific age ranges assessed as part of age-specific competencies.

- **Identify the objectives that must be achieved to demonstrate competency.** These objectives should be written in measurable terms and contain action verbs such as "performs," "identifies," "demonstrates," etc. Nonmeasurable terms such as "understand," "be aware of," etc., are to be avoided.

- **Document specific steps in competency achievement.** Consistency cannot be ensured unless the specific, step-by-step actions that must be performed to achieve competency are in writing. All assessors must have the same expectations of the people they are evaluating.

- **Document the methods used to assess competency.** Possible methods include observation of direct patient care, medical record review, and evaluation of the patient's environment. Again, don't forget to identify what the assessor must look for in the selected method(s).

- **Document remedial action.** If competency is not achieved, document the remedial actions that will be taken to help the learner achieve competency. The actions should be specific and include target achievement dates.

Conclusion

Competency assessment is an integral part of your patient care delivery system. Those who assess the competency of others must receive appropriate education and training so that they are effective, efficient, and consistent in their approach.

Careful, objective documentation of such education and training is as important as documentation of competency assessment itself. In fact, achievement as a competency assessor is a competency too. Select those individuals who assess competency with care. Not every staff member is suited to assess and facilitate learning in others. Clinical excellence does not equate with the ability to facilitate the job performance of colleagues.

The templates and forms presented in this chapter are intended to be starting points for the customization of your own tools. Adapt them to meet the needs of your staff members.

Finally, remember that competency assessment is a learning tool as well as a means of validation. Use these opportunities to facilitate the continuing education and professional development of staff members with the ultimate goal being improved patient outcomes.

References

Avillion, Adrianne E. *A Practical Guide to Staff Development: Tools and Techniques for Effective Education.* Marblehead, MA: HCPro, Inc., 2004.

Avillion, Adrianne E. *Age-Specific Care Training Handbook for Nurses and Clinical Care Staff.* Marblehead, MA: HCPro, Inc., 2004.

Bland, Gayle, and Lynn C. Hadaway. "Principles of adult learning." In Adrianne E. Avillion, ed. *Core Curriculum for Staff Development*, 2nd ed. Pensacola, FL: National Nursing Staff Development Organization, 2001. 31–64.

Chapter 5

Keep up with new competencies

CHAPTER 5

Keep up with new competencies

There are hundreds of new concerns arising in healthcare daily. How do you determine which become competencies?

Let's start by describing what a competency is not. Competencies are not required for every new piece of equipment, every new or revised policy and procedure, every interpersonal communication problem, or every skill that accompanies a specific job description. However, a competency is a skill that significantly affects or has the potential to significantly affect the patient. Such issues may fall under the categories of psychomotor skills or interpersonal skills.

Doesn't everything in healthcare have the potential to significantly affect a patient? Technically, yes. But if you define the word "significant" that broadly, you will have so many competencies that you'll drown in paperwork, and it will become impossible to assess that many items efficiently.

Potential categories for new competencies

Let's look at some general categories that have the potential for competency development.

New equipment

Not every piece of new equipment triggers the need for a competency. In most cases, a simple inservice suffices. For example, suppose your organization orders new patient beds. The beds have some additional features that the old beds lacked, and an inservice is conducted to orient staff to work safely with these new beds. Now suppose that new equipment including Circoelectric beds, Bradford frames, and Stryker frames arrive for your organization's newly opened rehabilitation unit. These devices require special skills to ensure patient safety and will be used often, although not daily. These types of new equipment are more suitable for ongoing competency development. They have significant patient impact, require a high level of skill and safety awareness, and are in frequent use.

When new equipment arrives, ask yourself these questions:

1. Does the equipment require high levels of skill to operate?

2. Who will operate the new equipment? Must staff have special qualifications (e.g., registered nurse) to use this equipment?

3. What potential patient safety risks are associated with the new equipment?

4. How often will the new equipment be in use?

If you find that equipment requires qualified staff members to have high levels of skill, is associated with significant patient safety issues, and is used often enough that staff are able to maintain competency, then the equipment may require the development of a competency.

Interpersonal communications

Interpersonal communications are the foundation of healthcare interventions. From the first contact at a reception desk or admission's office through and including communication with physicians, nurses, and therapists, interpersonal interaction influences the patient's healthcare experience.

How would you rate interpersonal communication skills among your colleagues? Does risk management/quality improvement data indicate any negative trends in this arena? Do staff members encounter hostility from patients/families? This is not uncommon, especially in areas such as the emergency department, head trauma unit, and inpatient mental health unit. But how do you assess this type of competency? It is not a step-by-step psychomotor skill. However, there are options.

Direct observation is one such option. Keep in mind, however, that written guidelines are necessary for the person assessing competency. Additional observations may be set up in a "competency skills lab" where staff must respond to various types of behavior in role-play situations. These are not conducted in the actual work setting, but they may be a useful addendum to direct observation.

Be creative when assessing nontechnical skills like these. Another validation option is to conduct mock drills involving staff members playing the role of agitated/violent patients or family members. These have the advantage of surprise and may be more valuable than a controlled role-play situation.

New patient populations

The appearance of new diseases and syndromes requires the implementation of new diagnostic and treatment interventions. The AIDS epidemic changed almost every aspect of healthcare and triggered the need for universal precautions and more secure protective equipment. The development of new drugs to combat this syndrome requires that healthcare professionals add to the ever-growing body of knowledge concerning medications, their actions, and potential side effects. Similarly, until recently, few healthcare professionals had ever heard of severe acute respiratory syndrome (SARS). Now it is a household name.

The point is that new patient populations require new knowledge and the application of that knowledge in the healthcare setting. As you evaluate the need for new skills to apply this knowledge, you are also evaluating the need for additional competency development. However, stick to the recommendations made earlier in this chapter. Consider the level of knowledge and skill needed, how often the knowledge will be applied, and the effect of these newly acquired skills on patient outcomes.

New treatment measures

Thanks to intense research and scientific inquiry, we are able to treat and even cure illnesses and catastrophic injuries that were untreatable even a few short years ago. With these healthcare advances come new bodies of knowledge and the need to use that knowledge safely and efficiently. As new treatment measures become necessary to your organization's ability to provide patient services, so does the need for additional competency development.

Remember that you don't need to keep the same competencies forever. Perhaps new treatments and equipment and the demise or reduction of certain illnesses (e.g., polio) trigger the need for you to delete certain competencies from your program. As you evaluate the need for new competencies, don't forget to evaluate the need to streamline those already in existence.

New medications

Significant numbers of new medications are approved annually by the Food and Drug Administration. Most of them do not require competency development; however, some drugs require special knowledge and administration techniques necessitate competency development. Use your guidelines of skill level, patient impact, and frequency of use to determine the need for new competencies.

Research endeavors

If your organization is a research site, your staff members may be exposed to new (and sometimes dangerous) ways of treating illnesses and injuries more often than the average healthcare worker. Examine your research policies and procedures. Which staff members frequently initiate experimental treatments, including medication administration? How do you measure their competency to initiate these treatments? As you evaluate your competency assessment program, don't forget to pay close attention to the research conducted at your organization: The resulting treatment initiatives could mandate the development of new competencies.

Guidelines for new competency development

Develop a policy that guides your competency assessment program. Part of that policy describes your guidelines for new competency development (and for the deletion of competencies that are no longer necessary).

Answer the following questions to identify what to incorporate into your organization's policy:

1. What new diagnostic tests, treatments, or other factors are developed that require staff members to add to their knowledge and expertise?

2. What current competencies no longer meet the criteria for ongoing competency assessment? Are the treatments outdated, are they no longer initiated, or have they become part of a daily routine with reduced impact on patient outcome and little or no exceptional level of skill?

3. What level of skill do new initiatives require?

4. Who is authorized to perform/evaluate the effectiveness of new initiatives?

5. What safety risks (to patients, visitors, and staff members) are associated with these new initiatives?

6. How often will these new initiatives be implemented?

Think about your answer to question number six carefully. Staff members cannot achieve or retain competency unless they have fairly regular opportunities to use new knowledge and skills. Consider the following example:

A newly opened, freestanding 100-bed rehabilitation facility does not have 24-hour physician coverage on-site. The patient population consists primarily of spinal-cord injury, stroke, traumatic head injury, hip fracture, multiple fracture, and amputee patients. Although the patients are relatively stable prior to their transfer to the facility, occasionally a patient deteriorates rapidly and emergency medical services (EMS) is notified. Patients also go into cardiac arrest. All direct patient care providers are cardiopulmonary resuscitation (CPR)-certified. In the event of cardiac arrest, CPR is initiated and an IV is started, and the use of a portable defibrillator is sanctioned if warranted. This procedure was developed with the assistance of EMS personnel. The arrival of the EMS squad from the local acute care health system takes between seven and 10 minutes.

The administrative staff (chief executive officer, director of nursing, and comptroller) expressed concern that patients could not be intubated and advance life support drugs administered prior to the arrival of the EMS squad. They decided to mandate that all registered nurses (RN) working at the rehabilitation facility achieve and maintain advanced cardiac life support (ACLS) certification.

Chapter 5—Keep up with new competencies

These nurses, on the rare occasion of a cardiac arrest, would be expected to intubate patients and initiate ACLS treatment measures, including the administration of cardiac medications. The RNs would need to demonstrate ongoing competency in ACLS to keep their jobs. Is this a realistic competency?

The answer, of course, is no. Nurses cannot maintain competency in a procedure as complex as ACLS when they do not have regular opportunities to use such knowledge and skills. In fact, attempting to intubate a patient when you only have an opportunity to do so once a year is extremely dangerous.

The EMS representatives teamed up with the facility's staff development specialists to convince the administrative staff that attempting to mandate ACLS certification would do more harm than good. But until this was accomplished, the nursing staff were quite upset, and some even resigned rather than attempt to achieve ACLS certification.

This example illustrates the importance of being able to use knowledge and apply skills to achieve and maintain competency. Knowledge acquisition alone is not enough.

The following checklist may help you to document your assessment of the need for new competency development.

Figure 5.1 — New competency assessment checklist

Date: _____

Item being evaluated:
- ☐ New equipment
- ☐ New treatment
- ☐ New medication
- ☐ New patient population
- ☐ Interpersonal communication issue
- ☐ Research initiatives

Identify the item specifically (e.g., type and purpose of equipment, description of new treatment, etc.).

_____
_____
_____

1. What new knowledge/skills are required to safely initiate this new item?

_____
_____
_____

2. Who is authorized to perform these new skills? (e.g., RNs, LPNs, etc.)

_____
_____
_____

3. What, if any, quality improvement/risk management data indicate a need for this competency?

_____
_____
_____

4. What risks to patients, visitors, and staff members are associated with the new initiative?

_____
_____
_____

> **Figure 5.1** **New competency assessment checklist (cont.)**

5. How often will staff members have an opportunity to apply the new knowledge and skills necessary for safe, accurate implementation of this new initiative?

_____
_____
_____

There is a need for new competency development. The new competency is:

_____
_____
_____

_____

Signature, title, and date

There is no need for new competency development. The rationale for this is:

_____
_____
_____

_____

Signature, title, and date

Best practices for the implementation of new competencies

Unfortunately, new competencies do not evolve neatly on an annual basis, allowing ample time for appropriate education and training to occur. They pop up at any time, with varying degrees of urgency. Here are some suggestions for implementation of new competencies.

Competency skills fairs

Some organizations have implemented day-long or half-day competency-assessment days. These are called by various names, such as "skill fairs," "competency days," "competency skills labs," etc. The premise is generally the same: A variety of competencies are assessed during a specified time period and at an identified general location (usually a classroom setting). These events can be held at specified times throughout the year, such as annually, semiannually, or quarterly.

Advantages of this approach include the following:

1. Efficiency. Competency days allow you to address the maximum number of people with a minimum number of observers.

2. Regular scheduling. Staff members know when these events will occur and, in conjunction with their managers, can plan their attendance. Likewise, persons responsible for organizing the competency days have planning time and the chance to add/delete competencies.

3. Decreased time away from the actual work site. By planning regular assessment days, staffing needs can be planned in advance.

Disadvantages of this approach include the following:

1. Competencies are only added or deleted at specific times throughout the year. This may compromise the timeliness of critical competency assessments.

2. Competencies that require demonstration of actual patient care interactions/procedures are not suitable for this approach.

3. Having sufficient competency assessors on hand can be problematic.

4. The length of time the fair is open can be a challenge. Twenty-four-hour availability requires a large number of competency assessors. If 24-hour availability is not possible, determining the hours of operation can draw complaints from staff who must attend on their off time. In addition, because competency assessment is a mandate, staff members are entitled to be paid for attending these types of events, which can place a considerable burden on the organization's budget.

Drills and simulations

An evaluation form must be completed after each drill. This form serves as a record of behavior, a competency assessment, and a format to document strengths and areas for improvement. Examples of drills and simulations include mock codes, internal and external disasters, and hazardous spill clean-up.

Drills and simulations

1. require little or no additional staffing

2. can serve as a complement to the annual review of the environment of care plans required by the Occupational Safety and Health Administration

3. evaluate behavior in true-to-life situations

Disadvantages of drills and simulations are that they

1. may disrupt other programs or patient care activities

2. require exceptionally well-qualified evaluators

3. need specific identification of required behaviors on evaluation forms

Performance improvement monitors

This approach relies on data from performance improvement (PI) documentation. PI indicators are useful when evaluating both interpersonal competencies and abilities to perform clinical skills.

Advantages of using PI monitors include the following:

1. It is a regular, reliable source of data

2. There is no additional time burden required to collect the data

3. Mangers can simultaneously validate competency and complete a mandated activity without additional work, making the process more efficient

Disadvantages of using PI monitors include the following:

1. They require the assumption that the PI data is accurate and objective

2. They do not guarantee that competency was consistently evaluated if multiple persons had input into the performance evaluation

Return demonstration/observation

Return demonstration can take place during the previously mentioned skills fair or on the job, which involves direct observation of skill performance.

Return demonstration/observation

1. allows the assessor to actually see behavior and the employee's application of knowledge

2. allows for demonstration of new knowledge and skills in the actual work environment in "real-life" settings

Disadvantages of return demonstration/observation include the following:

1. May influence the behavior of the staff member being assessed because he or she is aware that an evaluation is taking place

2. Cannot guarantee that employees' behavior is the same during the return demonstration/observation as when not being observed

Self-assessment

Self-assessment generally requires that employees complete a written exercise designed to identify the employees' beliefs and knowledge about their job performance. The employees' assessment is compared to the managers' and other assessors' assessments. Any disparity must be addressed so that job performance improves.

Self-assessment

1. helps employees recognize their own beliefs and values and how these issues may affect their job performance

2. identifies incongruence between employees' beliefs and values and the organization's mission, vision, and values

Disadvantages of self-assessment include the following:

1. It does not provide an opportunity for evaluation of the actual behaviors

2. Results are influenced by employees' and assessors' personal values and beliefs

3. Failure to address incongruence results in employees' continuing to behave in ways that are inconsistent with the organization's mission, vision, and values

Dimensions of competencies

Each approach is distinct and focuses on specific aspects of employee skills. According to Joan Tracy and Brenda Summers in *Competency Assessment: A Practical Guide to the JCAHO Standards*, competencies are designed to evaluate particular features of skills, called dimensions. Each dimension includes explicit skills and knowledge. They include the following:

- *Critical thinking dimension*: The ability to use information or knowledge, including

    - problem solving
    - planning
    - clinical reasoning
    - adapting/facilitating change
    - time management
    - fiscal responsibility

- *Interpersonal dimension*: The ability to work effectively with others, including

    - communication
    - conflict management
    - customer service
    - working effectively with members of various cultures and racial and ethnic backgrounds
    - working as effective team players

- *Technical dimension*: The possession of knowledge and the ability to use that knowledge to perform fine and gross motor functions, including

    - cognitive abilities
    - acquired knowledge
    - psychomotor ability
    - technical competence

As you evaluate the need for new competencies, review these dimensions to determine both need and approach. Remember that a competency assessment program focuses on verifying and validating skills and knowledge application in the work place. The purpose of a competency program is to

- improve job performance
- enhance patient outcomes
- promote economic efficiency
- increase organizational effectiveness

Demonstrated achievement of these goals shows that your competency assessment program is one that not only validates knowledge and skills but also results in improved patient outcomes.

References

Avillion, Adrianne E. *A Practical Guide to Staff Development: Tools and Techniques for Effective Education*. Marblehead, MA: HCPro, Inc., 2004.

Tracy, Joan, and Brenda Summers. *Competency Assessment: A Practical Guide to the JCAHO Standards*. Marblehead, MA: HCPro, Inc., 2001.

Chapter 6

Using your skills checklists

Chapter 6

Using your skills checklists

Skills checklists must clearly identify expectations and should be completed by staff members who know how to use them. Criteria for safe, effective performance must be clearly defined, and everyone participating in the evaluation process must have a common understanding of the criteria and the basis for assigning ratings. Research has shown that if evaluators make direct observations using precise measurement criteria in checklists, with immediate feedback on performance, this is more effective than the traditional evaluation of clinical skills using subjective rating forms. The format for skills checklists may vary, but most contain similar information. Regardless of how they are used, skills checklists should

- be learner-oriented
- focus on behaviors
- be measurable
- use criteria validated by experts
- be specific enough to avoid ambiguity

A template used to create the skills checklists included in this book appears in Figure 6.1, and an electronic version of this template appears on your CD-ROM. It can be opened as a Microsoft Word document. For instructions on how to download the template, see p. 109. The individual's name and date are important to identify whose skills are being validated and when it is being done.

Figure 6.1: Skills checklist template

Name: _____ Date: _____

Skill: _____

Steps	Completed	Comments

Self-assessment	Evaluation/validation methods	Levels	Type of validation	Comments
☐ Experienced ☐ Need practice ☐ Never done ☐ Not applicable (based on scope of practice)	☐ Verbal ☐ Demonstration/observation ☐ Practical exercise ☐ Interactive class	☐ Beginner ☐ Intermediate ☐ Expert	☐ Orientation ☐ Annual ☐ Other _____	

_____   _____
Employee signature   **Observer signature**

The steps identified in the checklist should define the critical behaviors needed for effective performance of the skill and do not include every step of the procedure. The completed column can be used to indicate that each step was performed correctly; some checklists use a met/not met format. It is helpful if checklists include an area for comments, and most checklists are used to evaluate a single occurrence.

In the checklist format given on p. 84, the self-assessment can give the evaluator an idea of the perceived skill level of the individual, although that can never take the place of validating competency. Individuals may have different perceptions of their abilities that may or may not be consistent with the evaluator's perceptions. For instance, one person could indicate that he or she needs practice, even though that person is familiar and competent with that skill, but he or she is not familiar with the institution's policy and procedure. Another staff member could indicate that he or she needs practice because the staff member has only performed it once during their career. All required skills must be validated, regardless of the individual's assessment of his or her ability.

The evaluation/validation methods areas indicate how the validation was done. The method used most often is demonstration or observation of the individual performing the skill, but verbal questioning can also be effective in identifying the thought processes or critical thinking involved with skills. Practical exercises and interactive class activities can also be useful as validation methods.

The appropriate level (beginner, intermediate, or expert) can be indicated, as well as the type of validation. It is important to identify whether the assessment is part of an individual's orientation or ongoing annual validation and to have both the employee and observer sign the checklist. The Joint Commission on Accreditation of Healthcare Organizations (JCAHO) mandates that all employees have their competence assessed upon hire and throughout their employment. One way to meet this standard is to have orientation checklists in addition to skills checklists.[1]

Difference between orientation checklists and skills checklists

Orientation checklists specify knowledge, attitudes, and skills needed to perform safely. The information for an orientation checklist would come from the position description for that job classification and would outline the essential competencies for safe practice in that role. Skills checklists,

Chapter 6—Using your skills checklists

on the other hand, include the specific tasks related to a policy or procedure. Skills checklists are often used to document ongoing competency, as compared to orientation checklists, which document initial competency.

Developing orientation checklists

Key elements in developing an orientation checklist are the job description and performance evaluation criteria. The components of the orientation program provide the framework. Essential information in the checklist would include the individual's name and the names of all evaluators. Hire date and unit are helpful to identify when the individual started in his or her role. Orientation checklists provide documentation of the initial assessment of competence required by JCAHO, as well as the individual's self-assessment. If evaluation during the orientation is a shared responsibility (e.g., with staff development educators and unit preceptors), different columns can be used to identify what was done during a classroom orientation and what was done in the clinical area. A "not evaluated" or "not applicable" column can be helpful for those skills that an orientee did not have an opportunity to perform during the orientation process.

Sample checklists for registered nurse (RN) orientation (Figure 6.2) and nursing assistant (NA) orientation (Figure 6.3) are included as examples.

Orientation checklists should be developed with input from the management staff. This will ensure that they include the essential skills expected from the position. Generally, staff development personnel/preceptors complete orientation checklists. Preceptors help new employees adjust to the workplace and clinical unit and work with new employees to help plan the learning experiences and share knowledge of expected behaviors. They can help reduce stress and enhance learning for new employees by using adult learning principles, documenting skill acquisition, and helping the new person socialize into the unit culture. The checklist helps make employees accountable for their learning by clearly identifying expectations to be completed during the orientation period. After the orientation checklist is completed, it usually becomes part of the employee's permanent file, which protects both the employer and the employee.

Figure 6.2 — Competency-based orientation checklist

SUMMA HEALTH SYSTEM STAFF DEVELOPMENT
RN Skills Assessment/Evaluation

Name: _____   Hire Date: _____
Unit: _____

Staff Development: Initials: Preceptors: Initials:

_____   _____   _____   _____
_____   _____   _____   _____
_____   _____   _____   _____
_____   _____
_____

Directions:

Orientee: Complete the self assessment by placing a check (✓) in the appropriate column based on your level of familiarity or experience with each competency.

Staff Development/Preceptor: Complete the evaluation section for each competency after the orientee has demonstrated successful completion of that competency. Place the date and your initials in the appropriate column. If NE (not evaluated) is checked, include an explanation in the comments column.

	SELF ASSESSMENT			EVALUATION			
Competencies	Comfortable	Need review	Have never done	*SD ORT	Unit	**NE	Comments
I. COMPETENCY **A. Applies a systematic problem-solving approach in the implementation of nursing plans of care:**							
1. Uses nursing process to systematically assess, plan, implement and evaluate nursing care.							
2. Provide/documents patient teaching/discharge planning.							

*SD ORT = Staff Development Orientation   **NE = If Not Evaluated, indicate explanation

Figure 6.2 Competency-based orientation checklist (cont.)

Competencies	SELF ASSESSMENT			EVALUATION			
	Comfortable	Need review	Have never done	*SD ORT	Unit	**NE	Comments
3. Involves patient/significant other in plan of care.							
4. Prioritizes nursing care for a group of patients.							
5. Initiates patient referrals as needed.							
6. Utilizes appropriate resources.							
B. Intravenous therapy							
1. Initiates IV							
2. Monitors IV according to policy and procedure a. Checks rate							
b. Assesses for signs and symptoms of complications							
c. Initiates PRN adapter							
3. Uses infusion pumps correctly: • PCA							
• Baxter							
4. Draws blood specimens: • Routine							
• Central line							
• Blood cultures							
5. Administers blood and blood components.							
6. Maintains central line/hyperalimentation.							
7. Applies/changes central line dressing.							

*SD ORT = Staff Development Orientation   **NE = If Not Evaluated, indicate explanation

CHAPTER 6—USING YOUR SKILLS CHECKLISTS

Figure 6.2 Competency-based orientation checklist (cont.)

Competencies	SELF ASSESSMENT			EVALUATION			
	Comfortable	Need review	Have never done	*SD ORT	Unit	**NE	Comments
8. Administers IV medications (IVPB, IV push).							
9. Documents administration of IV therapy.							
10. Completes IV therapy exam with a minimum score of 80%.							
C. Medication administration							
1. Describes usual dose, common side effects, compatibilities, action, and untoward reactions to medications.							
2. Administers medications: a. Intramuscular							
b. Subcutaneous and insulin							
c. Calculations							
d. Other							
3. Documents administration of medications (MAR, controlled drugs, etc.).							
4. Identifies medication error reporting system.							
D. Treatment and procedures							
1. Inserts and maintains gastric feeding tubes.							
2. Inserts and maintains urinary catheters.							
3. Performs trach care and suctioning.							

*SD ORT = Staff Development Orientation   **NE = If Not Evaluated, indicate explanation

COMPETENCY MANAGEMENT FOR THE EMERGENCY DEPARTMENT

Figure 6.2 Competency-based orientation checklist (cont.)

Competencies	SELF ASSESSMENT			EVALUATION			
	Comfortable	Need review	Have never done	*SD ORT	Unit	**NE	Comments
4. Assesses patient safety including proper utilization of restraints.							
5. Completes tissue therapy self-learning packet (SLP)							
6. Provides and documents pre and post-op nursing care.							
7. Incorporates nursing measures to reduce and prevent the spread of infection in daily nursing care.							
8. Completes American Heart Association guidelines for BLS/CPR.							
9. Changes oxygen gauge sets rate.							
10. Locates various items on the emergency cart.							
11. Identifies nursing responsibilities in emergency situations.							
12. Completes a. Admission of patient							
b. Transfer of a patient.							
c. Discharge of a patient.							
13. Performs neurological checks when appropriate.							
14. Performs blood-glucose test.							
15. Other.							

*SD ORT = Staff Development Orientation   **NE = If Not Evaluated, indicate explanation

Figure 6.2 Competency-based orientation checklist (cont.)

Competencies	SELF ASSESSMENT			EVALUATION			
	Comfortable	Need review	Have never done	*SD ORT	Unit	**NE	Comments
II. COMMUNICATION A. Documents on the following forms: • Initial interdisciplinary assessment							
• Graphic record							
• Interdisciplinary progress record							
• Nursing discharge/ patient teaching							
• Interdisciplinary plan of care							
• Unusual occurrence							
B. Transcribes physician's orders.							
C. Takes verbal orders from physician.							
D. Uses correct lines of communication.							
E. Attends computer class.							
F. Gives prompt, accurate, and pertinent shift report.							
G. Interacts with patients, significant others, and health team members in a positive manner.							
III. ACCOUNTABILITY/ LEADERSHIP A. Completes orientation statement of agreement.							

*SD ORT = Staff Development Orientation **NE = If Not Evaluated, indicate explanation

Figure 6.2 **Competency-based orientation checklist (cont.)**

Competencies	SELF ASSESSMENT			EVALUATION			
	Comfortable	Need review	Have never done	*SD ORT	Unit	**NE	Comments
B. Delegates patient care to other personnel appropriately.							
C. Follows appropriate employee policies and procedures (i.e., call off, time off, leave of absence, etc.).							
D. Conforms to dress code.							
E. Identifies role of the nurse in quality assurance.							
F. Maintains safe working environment.							
G. Contains costs through proper use of supplies and maintenance of equipment.							
IV. OTHER: A. Has completed human resource/safety orientation.							

RELEASE FROM ORIENTATION

The undersigned employee/orientee can be released from orientation as of _____ (date).

_____   _____   _____
Orientee Signature   Preceptor Signature   Unit Manager Signature

Return this form and orientation paperwork/folder to ACH Nursing Records or STMC Human Resources when completed.

Skills still needing supervision are listed below. It is the responsibility of the employee/orientee to be supervised prior to performing these skills: _____

_____

*SD ORT = Staff Development Orientation   **NE = If Not Evaluated, indicate explanation

Source: Summa Health System Hospitals, Akron, OH. Reprinted with permission.

CHAPTER 6—USING YOUR SKILLS CHECKLISTS

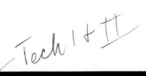

Figure 6.3 — Nursing assistant orientation checklist

SUMMA HEALTH SYSTEM HOSPITALS
STAFF DEVELOPMENT

COMPETENCY-BASED CHECKLIST

NURSING ASSISTANT ORIENTATION
SKILLS ASSESSMENT/EVALUATION

NAME: _____

HIRE DATE (this role): _____

UNIT: _____

STAFF DEVELOPMENT: _____ INITIALS: _____

PRECEPTORS: _____ INITIALS: _____

Directions:

Orientee:
Complete the self assessment by placing a check (✓) in the appropriate column based on your level of familiarity or experience with each competency.

Staff Development/Preceptor:
Complete the evaluation section for each competency after the orientee has demonstrated successful completion of that competency. Place the date and your initials in the appropriate column. If NE (not evaluated) is checked, include an explanation in the comments column.

Competencies	SELF ASSESSMENT			EVALUATION			
	Comfortable	Need review	Have Never done	Date Met Initials *SD ORT	Unit	** NE	Comments
A. Demonstrates ability to do basic patient care as follows:							
1. Complete bed bath							
2. Partial bath							
3. Assists with shower							
4. Oral Hygiene							
5. Back care							
6. Peri care							
7. Hair care							
8. Offering/removal of bed pan/urinal							
9. Cath care							
10. Documentation of output on Kardex or worksheet							Unit based competency on file.

*SD ORT = Staff Development Orientation   **NE = If Not Evaluated, indicate explanation

COMPETENCY MANAGEMENT FOR THE EMERGENCY DEPARTMENT

Figure 6.3 Nursing assistant orientation checklist (cont.)

Competencies	SELF ASSESSMENT			EVALUATION			
	Comfortable	Need review	Have Never done	Date Met Initials		**NE	Comments
				*SD ORT	Unit		
A. Demonstrates ability to do basic patient care as follows: *(Continued)* 11. Feeding of patient, including compensatory strategies for feeding dysphagic patient							
12. Shaving of patient							
13. Occupied bed							
14. Unoccupied bed							
15. Accurately measuring patient intake and output and recording on appropriate form							
16. Patient transfer/ discharge							
17. Pneumatic Cuffs							
18. K-Pad							
B. Body Mechanics 1. Discusses the proper techniques of lifting/ turning/transferring patient							
2. Demonstrates proper technique in transferring patient from bed to cart and back							
3. Demonstrates proper technique transferring patient from bed to wheelchair							
4. Demonstrates proper technique in positioning and turning patients							
C. Technical Skills 1. Assesses patient safety including proper utilization and documentation of restraints							

*SD ORT = Staff Development Orientation   **NE = If Not Evaluated, indicate explanation

Figure 6.3 — Nursing assistant orientation checklist (cont.)

Competencies	SELF ASSESSMENT			EVALUATION			
	Comfortable	Need review	Have Never done	Date Met Initials *SD ORT	Unit	** NE	Comments
C. Technical Skills *(Continued)*							
2. Completes American Heart Association guidelines for Heartsaver Course				----			
3. Monitors oxygen tank gauge				----			
4. Identifies responsibilities in emergency situations							
5. Incorporates measures to reduce and prevent the spread of infection in daily patient care							
D. Demonstrates ability to take and record vital signs. Temperature:							Unit based competency checklist on file.
1. Takes oral temperature and records							
2. Discusses procedure for rectal temperature				----			
Radial pulse:							
1. Counts and records pulse rate							
Respirations:							
1. Counts respiratory rate and records							
E. Demonstrates ability to obtain and transport appropriately the following specimens:							
1. Sputum							
2. Urine/routine/ccms							
3. Stool							
4. Blood, transport only							

*SD ORT = Staff Development Orientation   **NE = If Not Evaluated, indicate explanation

Figure 6.3 Nursing assistant orientation checklist (cont.)

Competencies	SELF ASSESSMENT			EVALUATION			
	Comfortable	Need review	Have Never done	Date Met Initials *SD ORT	Unit	** NE	Comments
F. Performs post mortem care							
G. Transports patient to morgue							
H. Removes dirty linen or equipment from patient room							
I. Passes and picks up trays							
1. Records Intake (and output) accurately on worksheet in room.							Unit based competency checklist on file.
2. Empty and replace trash bags, remove excess linen, etc., from patient rooms,							
K. Maintenance needs:							
1. Verbalizes safety issues with equipment (step ladders, hand tools, light bulbs, etc.)							
2. Identifies light maintenance duties							
L. Demonstrates ability to Assess Just-In-Time technician. (Distribution)							
M. Demonstrates proper use of communication:							Unit based competency checklist on file.
1. Patient Intercom							
2. Answering patient call light							
3. Telephone/answering phone appropriately by identifying unit, name, and status							
4. Operating pneumatic tube system, describe purpose and use							

*SD ORT = Staff Development Orientation   **NE = If Not Evaluated, indicate explanation

Figure 6.3 — Nursing assistant orientation checklist (cont.)

Competencies	SELF ASSESSMENT			EVALUATION			
	Comfortable	Need review	Have Never done	Date Met Initials *SD ORT	Unit	**NE	Comments
5. Explaining the importance of patient confidentiality							
6. Communicating to R.N. any unusual observations (Signs and Symptoms)							
N. Interacts with patients, significant others, and health team members in positive manner.							
O. Safety Issues: (Each orientee should be able to discuss and correctly answer questions on the following safety topics)							
1. Fire Safety (Code Red)				----			
2. Bomb Threat (Code Black)				----			
3. Code Violet				----			
4. Infection Prevention and Exposure Control				----			
5. Disaster (Code Yellow)				----			
6. Evacuation				----			
7. Back Safety				----			
8. Severe Weather				----			
9. Electrical Safety				----			
10. Code Adam				----			
P. Punctuality:							
1. Arrives on unit in uniform on time							
2. Notifies nursing office of absence according to policy							
3. Notifies nursing office of lateness according to policy							
4. Notifies nurse in charge when leaving unit and reason							

*SD ORT = Staff Development Orientation   **NE = If Not Evaluated, indicate explanation

Figure 6.3 — Nursing assistant orientation checklist (cont.)

Competencies	SELF ASSESSMENT			EVALUATION			
	Comfortable	Need review	Have Never done	Date Met Initials *SD ORT	Unit	**NE	Comments
5. Follows current hospital guidelines for breaks and lunch hours							
6. Returns from errands and meetings promptly							
Q. Examinations: Completes the following exams with a minimum score of 70%:							
1. Medical Abbreviation Test				----			
2. Patient Safety Test				----			
3. Patient Limited Activity Test				----			
4. Grooming and Oral Hygiene Test				----			
R. Other:							

*SD ORT = Staff Development Orientation   **NE = If Not Evaluated, indicate explanation

Source: Summa Health System Hospitals, Akron, OH. Reprinted with permission.

Skills checklists for annual competency assessment

This section will provide suggestions on how to determine what skills to evaluate, develop the skills checklists, identify who can complete the checklists, and keep track of who has been evaluated. It will also review what happens if someone does not meet identified competencies and include a brief discussion of other methods of validating competence.

Determining what skills to evaluate

Your organization needs to set up a system to determine which competencies to evaluate each year. A suggested formula to use when determining which skills to evaluate was provided in Chapter 2. There is no right or wrong way to select what skills will be evaluated, as long as the organization can justify why the particular skills were chosen. Skills should be selected based on the individual needs of the unit or organization.

Developing the skills checklists

Once the skills to be assessed are selected, skill checklists can be developed or modified from the samples attached to ensure consistency in evaluation. Review your institution's policies and procedures using current literature for support. The essential steps of the policy and procedure are incorporated into the skills checklists, many of which can easily be adapted for your institution by changing the criteria to be consistent with steps in your policies and procedures or standards.

Identifying who can complete the checklists

It is important to identify who (e.g., what job classification) can validate skills for each job classification. It may be better to have a RN or LPN check off an NA on vital signs rather than to have another NA complete the skills checklist. Individuals who are responsible to validate someone's skill should be qualified by education, experience, or expertise with that skill, or they should have already demonstrated proficiency with that skill. An individual with documented competence in that skill should assess ongoing competence. That competence may be determined by his or her role (e.g., advanced practice nurse, staff development instructor, unit managers, specialist coordinator, etc.), frequency of performing the skill, or already having demonstrated competence in that skill.

When introducing new technology or procedures into the clinical area, the initial training should be done by individuals with documented experience in that procedure (e.g., physician, nurses from that specialty, vendor representatives, etc.). A core group of staff members or a single individual can be trained and confirm competency of other staff members after they personally demonstrate competence in that skill.

Keeping track of who has been evaluated

Each evaluator should refer to the skills checklist when observing a staff member perform that skill. Skills checklists for the competencies being evaluated can be kept in a competency notebook as a reference for staff. These checklists can be used to assess initial and ongoing competence. The use of a checklist ensures consistency in evaluating the steps to perform the skill. Rather than completing an individual skills checklist for every person evaluated, a tracking sheet can usually be used to document completion of that skill.

The tracking sheet provides a way to document that staff members in each classification have completed required competencies. Names of the unit personnel are written on the tracking sheet, and when someone is checked off on a particular competency, the individual observing them writes in the date and his or her initials in the column for that particular competency in the row with their name. Individuals are responsible to ensure that someone validates their required skills each year. The manager then uses this information when completing performance appraisals.

The Competencies Analyzer

A sample of a tracking sheet is provided in Figure 6.4. We've provided an electronic version of this Excel spreadsheet on your CD-ROM. The Competencies Analyzer is an easy way for a manager to track competency assessment on his or her unit.

For instructions on how to download the Competencies Analyzer, see p. 109.

Figure 6.4 — Competencies tracking sheet

SUMMA HEALTH SYSTEM HOSPITALS
UNIT BASED COMPETENCY CHECKLIST
Unit Secretary

MEDICAL SURGICAL UNIT: _____

EMPLOYEE NAME	SUMMA	DEPT	DIVISION	COMPETENCY VERIFIED — UNIT BASED													
	1. Mandatory Safety Education	2. Heart Saver	See schedule for Mandatory Ed. and SLPs														

Source: Summa Health System Hospitals, Akron, OH. Reprinted with permission.

Determining what happens when staff cannot perform competencies

Organizations need to identify the consequences when a staff member cannot demonstrate mastery of a competency. Policies may vary, but a mechanism needs to be in place to safeguard patients and ensure that the staff member is not assigned to a patient who requires that competency. Possible options would be to provide remediation and further clinical experiences or transfer the staff member to another area where he or she can meet the required competencies. Continued failure to demonstrate required competencies may lead to a plan for improvement or termination.

Other methods to validate competence

It is also important to realize that the skills checklists are only one method to validate competence; other methods may be used. Some skills may not happen frequently enough to check all staff members off on that skill, and skills fairs may be an alternative approach. During skills fairs, employees are tested and validated on skills using simulations, games, word puzzles, or other methods to verify that they are aware of the steps of the procedure. Skills checklists can also be used during fairs for those skills that may not come up frequently enough to check everyone on the unit.

With the increasing sophistication of technology, computer-assisted video evaluation may be used to evaluate competency in a particular area. Videotaped or simulated scenarios can give evaluators the opportunity to observe and rate performances. With this approach, ratings can be compared with the instructor to clarify any discrepancies and determine inter-rater reliability. However, this may not be realistic in organizations where there are many staff members who will be completing skills checklists for their peers.

One problem with skills checklists is that you don't know whether the observed behavior is persistent and representative of the situation being observed, or whether the individual is going through the correct steps knowing that someone is evaluating them for that single occurrence. Therefore, indirect observation can also be used. Often managers or charge nurses conduct patient rounds and medical record reviews. With indirect observation, there may not be direct observation of the skills, but there is the presumption that the skills are correctly followed when the desired outcomes are achieved. Clinical rounds can measure competencies as well as improve the standard of care and practice in the clinical setting.

Chapter 6—Using your skills checklists

Organizations need to have a competency-based program in place to ensure that individuals are prepared to deliver quality patient care. Assessment of competency begins with orientation and continues throughout employment. An evaluation of each nursing staff member's competency should be conducted at defined intervals throughout the individual's association with the organization. Performance appraisals and skills checklists may be used to measure ongoing competency of nursing employees. Continuing education programs and inservices can also enhance staff members' competency.

Competence assessment for nursing staff and volunteers who provide direct patient care is based on the following:

1. Populations served, including age ranges and specialties

2. Competencies required for role and provision of care

3. Competencies assessed during orientation

4. Unit-specific competencies that need to be assessed or reassessed on a year basis based on care modalities, age ranges, techniques, procedures, technology, equipment, skills needed, or changes in law and regulations

5. Appropriate assessment methods for the skill being assessed

6. Delineation of who is qualified to assess competence

7. Description of action taken when improvement activities lead to a determination that a staff member with performance problems is unable or unwilling to improve

Individuals who transfer from another area in the organization know what competencies they must meet at the time of their orientation.

Chapter 6—Using your skills checklists

Karen Kelly-Thomas, a recognized staff development expert, identified the following questions to be included in an evaluation of the competence assessment system:

1. Is new employee competence assessment completed during the initial orientation process?

2. Is employee orientation based on assessed competencies and the knowledge and skills required to deliver patient care services?

3. Is new employee competence assessment completed at the conclusion of the orientation process?

4. Do clinical staff participate in ongoing educational activities to acquire new competencies that support patient care delivery? Are those activities minimally based on quality improvement findings, new technology, therapeutic or pharmacology interventions, and learning needs of nursing staff?

5. Do management or leadership staff participate in competence assessment activities (i.e., clinical knowledge, skills, technology)?

6. Do management or leadership staff participate in ongoing education activities to acquire new competencies for patient care management (i.e., management development)?

7. Does the performance evaluation system address staff competence?

8. When competency deficiencies are noted, is there a plan for correction initiated and implemented?

9. Does reassessment of competence occur as necessary?

10. Are summaries of competence assessment findings available by individual, by patient care unit, and by department?

11. Are plans for competence maintenance and improvement documented?

12. Is an annual report submitted to the governing body?

13. Do policies and procedures exist to define the process of competence assessment?[2]

The overall competence assessment process must be reviewed on an ongoing basis to determine its effectiveness and any opportunities for improvement. This evaluation identifies what works, what doesn't, why it doesn't, and how it can be improved. It can take a very formal approach through survey methodology and interviews or a more informal approach of asking for subjective data and feedback from key people and groups.

References

1. Joint Commission on Accreditation of Healthcare Organizations. *Comprehensive accreditation manual for hospitals: The official handbook.* Oakbrook Terrace, IL: JCAHO, 2004.

2. Kelly-Thomas, Karen J. *Clinical and Nursing Staff Development: Current Competence, Future Focus.* 2nd ed. Philadelphia: Lippincott, 1998. 84.

How to use the files on your CD-ROM

The following file names correspond with tools listed in the book, *Competency Management for the Emergency Department*:

File name	Document
sstemp.rtf	Blank skillsheet template
analyze.xls	Competencies Analyzer

The following file names correspond with skills sheets listed in the Appendices:

ED — Emergency Department

File name	Document
ed1.rtf	12 Lead Electrode (Modified Limb Leads) Prep and Placement
ed2.rtf	Aircast Splint Application
ed3.rtf	Airway Management
ed4.rtf	Arterial Blood Gas (ABG) Interpretation
ed5.rtf	Brace Application—Ice Corset
ed6.rtf	Brace Application—L-S Corset
ed7.rtf	Brace Application—TLSO Brace
ed8.rtf	Bronchoscopy Set-up and Equipment Use
ed9.rtf	Buck's Traction
ed10.rtf	Contrast Reaction Management
ed11.rtf	Defibrillator Monitor (Heartstream XL)
ed12.rtf	Electrocardiogram (EKG) Interpretation
ed13.rtf	EKG, 12 Lead
ed14.rtf	Foreign Body Removal
ed15.rtf	Monitoring Lead Placement
ed16.rtf	Suture Set-Up
ed17.rtf	System 1000 Fluid Warmer—Level 1
ed18.rtf	Thermacyl Fluid Warmer

How to use the files on your CD-ROM

ed19.rtf	Thrombolytic Therapy
ed20.rtf	Tourniquet Safety
ed21.rtf	Triage—Diarrhea
ed22.rtf	Triage—Upper Respiratory Infection
ed23.rtf	Welch Allyn Ear Wash System
ed24.rtf	Women's Health Infant Safety Abduction Code Pink

ALL —(General, All Units)

File name	Document
all1.rtf	Accurate Pressure Measurements
all2.rtf	Age-Specific Competency Checklist RN-LPN
all3.rtf	Age-Specific Competency Checklist SA-AA
all4.rtf	Annual Competency Performance—Cleaning Delivery Rooms
all5.rtf	Annual Competency Performance—Quality of Instruction
all6.rtf	Blood Glucose Meter
all7.rtf	Blood Pressure Measurement
all8.rtf	Code Skills
all9.rtf	Emergency Preparedness
all10.rtf	Hand Washing
all11.rtf	Oximeter (Whole Blood O_2 Saturation)
all12.rtf	Oxygen Administration
all13.rtf	Telephone Skills
all14.rtf	Telephone Skills (Problem-Solving)
all15.rtf	Use Automated External Defibrillator (Heartstream FR2)

To adapt any of the files to your own facility, simply follow the instructions below to open the CD.

If you have trouble reading the forms, click on "View," and then "Normal." To adapt the forms, save them first to your own hard drive or disk (by clicking "File," then "Save as," and changing the system to your own). Then change the information enclosed in brackets to fit your facility, and add or delete any items that you wish to change.

Installation instructions

This product was designed for the Windows operating system and includes Microsoft Word files that will run under Windows 95/98 or greater. The CD will work on all PCs and most Macintosh systems. To run the files on the CD-ROM, take the following steps:

1. Insert the CD into your CD-ROM drive.

2. Double-click on the "My Computer" icon, next double-click on the CD drive icon.

3. Double-click on the files you wish to open.

4. Adapt the files by moving the cursor over the areas you wish to change, highlighting them, and typing in the new information using Microsoft Word.

5. To save a file to your facility's system, click on "File" and then click on "Save As." Select the location where you wish to save the file and then click on "Save."

6. To print a document, click on "File" and then click on "Print."

ED—Emergency Department

ED—Emergency Department

Contents

1. 12 Lead Electrode (Modified Limb Leads) Prep and Placement 113
2. Aircast Splint Application 114
3. Airway Management 115
4. Arterial Blood Gas (ABG) Interpretation 117
5. Brace Application — Ice Corset 118
6. Brace Application — L-S Corset 119
7. Brace Application — TLSO Brace 120
8. Bronchoscopy Set-up and Equipment Use 121
9. Buck's Traction 122
10. Contrast Reaction Management 123
11. Defibrillator Monitor (Heartstream XL) 125
12. Electrocardiogram (EKG) Interpretation 128
13. EKG, 12 Lead 129
14. Foreign Body Removal 131
15. Monitoring Lead Placement 132
16. Suture Set-Up 133
17. System 1000 Fluid Warmer — Level 1 134
18. Thermacyl Fluid Warmer 135
19. Thrombolytic Therapy 136
20. Tourniquet Safety 137
21. Triage — Diarrhea 138
22. Triage — Upper Respiratory Infection 139
23. Welch Allyn Ear Wash System 140
24. Women's Health Infant Safety Abduction Code Pink 142

ED—EMERGENCY DEPARTMENT

ok

Name: _____ Date: _____

Skill: | 12 Lead Electrode (Modified Limb Leads) Prep and Placement |

Steps	Completed	Comments
1. Prepares and organizes all materials prior to the test including: ETOH, nonsterile gauze, razor, adhesive tape, and electrode wires.		
2. Explains the procedure to the patient.		
3. Instructs the patient to disrobe to the waist.		
4. Shaves electrode sites clean with razor, PRN.		
5. Removes loose hairs with 3-in. adhesive tape, PRN.		
6. Thoroughly abrades electrode sites with ETOH-dampened nonsterile gauze.		
7. Locates and places electrodes at the correct anatomical positions. **Site Location** RA: at the concavity of the right lateral clavicle LA: at the concavity of the left lateral clavicle RL: on the rib cage at the right anterior axillary line LL: on the rib cage at the left anterior axillary line V1: right sternal border at the fourth intercostal space V2: left sternal border at the fourth intercostal space V3: on the transverse plane midway between V2 and V4 V4: fifth intercostals space at the right midclavicular Line V5: on a horizontal plane from V4, at the right anterior axillary line V6: on a horizontal plane for V4 and V5, at the right midaxillary line		

Self-assessment	Evaluation/validation methods	Levels	Type of validation	Comments
☐Experienced ☐Need practice ☐Never done ☐Not applicable (based on scope of practice)	☐Verbal ☐Demonstration/observation ☐Practical exercise ☐Interactive class	☐Beginner ☐Intermediate ☐Expert	☐Orientation ☐Annual ☐Other _____	

_____   _____
Employee signature   **Observer signature**

COMPETENCY MANAGEMENT FOR THE EMERGENCY DEPARTMENT

ED—EMERGENCY DEPARTMENT

OK

Name: _____ Date: _____

Skill: | Aircast Splint Application |

Steps	Completed	Comments
1. Verifies physician order for aircast splint application.		
2. Obtains and prepares brace (small, medium, or large). Unfastens straps, removes front panel, and opens the liner.		
3. Identifies patient and explains procedure.		
4. Places correct leg in the brace with heel seated against the back.		
5. Pulls linear forward (make sure to free any wrinkles).		
6. Wraps the liner around the leg then foot and secures the velcro.		
7. Positions the front panel and attaches straps from bottom to top.		
8. Tightens until snug and comfortable.		
9. To inflate, inserts bulb tip into valve and squeezes to desired compression level.		
10. If need to deflate, inserts other end of bulb (as marked) and deflates.		
11. Documents application on patient's chart.		
12. Makes appropriate charge on billing sheet.		

Self-assessment	Evaluation/validation methods	Levels	Type of validation	Comments
☐Experienced ☐Need practice ☐Never done ☐Not applicable (based on scope of practice)	☐Verbal ☐Demonstration/observation ☐Practical exercise ☐Interactive class	☐Beginner ☐Intermediate ☐Expert	☐Orientation ☐Annual ☐Other _____	

_____ _____
Employee signature   Observer signature

ED—EMERGENCY DEPARTMENT

Name: _____ Date: _____

Skill: Airway Management

Steps	Completed	Comments
A. Opens/maintains airway		
• Head tilt/chin lift.		
B. Airway adjuncts		
1. Inserts oral airway.		
2. Inserts nasopharyngeal airway.		
3. Applies mouth to mask and ventilates x3 breaths.		
4. Ventilates utilizing a bag-valve mask device x3 breaths.		
C. Endotracheal intubation		
1. Identifies principles of BSI and use of PPE.		
2. Prepares laryngoscope blade and handle.		
3. Verifies integrity of endotracheal tube cuff.		
4. Prepares stylet, if appropriate.		
5. Applies cricoid pressure, if appropriate.		
6. Inflates cuff when tube is in place.		
7. Verifies bilateral breath sounds.		
8. Oxygenates and ventilates via the endotracheal tube using the bag valve mask.		
9. Secures endotracheal tube.		
D. Endotracheal extubation		
1. Identifies principles of BSI and use of PPE.		
2. Describes extubation criteria: • V/S • ABGs • Secretion and airway control • Treatment of infection, disease process		

COMPETENCY MANAGEMENT FOR THE EMERGENCY DEPARTMENT

ED—Emergency Department

• Mental status • Nutritional status • Weaning parameters, T-piece trails • Documentation		
3. Raises head of bed.		
4. Hyperoxygenates /hyperventilates with at least three breaths/suction tube and oropharynx/hyperoxygenate.		
5. Attaches syringe.		
6. Cuts ties and/or tape.		
7. At peak inspiration, deflates cuff.		
8. Pulls tube out in one motion, on expiration.		
9. C & DB/suctions the oropharynx.		
10. Applies supplemental oxygen: • Nasal cannula • Face mask • Venturi mask • Nonrebreather mask.		
11. Assesses response.		
12. Identifies principles of disposal of infectious waste.		

Self-assessment	Evaluation/validation methods	Levels	Type of validation	Comments
☐Experienced ☐Need practice ☐Never done ☐Not applicable (based on scope of practice)	☐Verbal ☐Demonstration/observation ☐Practical exercise ☐Interactive class	☐Beginner ☐Intermediate ☐Expert	☐Orientation ☐Annual ☐Other _____	

_____   _____
Employee signature   **Observer signature**

ED—EMERGENCY DEPARTMENT

Name: _____ Date: _____

Skill: ABG Interpretation

Steps	Completed	Comments
1. Identifies whether the following values are abnormal from a patient's ABG report. • p^H • P_aCO_2 • P_aO_2 • S_aO_2 • HCO_3 • S_vO_2		
2. From the patient's ABG report, determines whether the following acid/base imbalances exist: • Respiratory acidosis • Respiratory alkalosis • Metabolic acidosis • Metabolic alkalosis • Mixed respiratory/metabolic acidosis or alkalosis.		
3. Correctly identifies one physical sign and symptom associated with the patient's ABG interpretation.		
4. Correctly identifies one intervention to assist the patient in returning to a normal acid/base balance.		
5. Makes appropriate referral to physician or respiratory therapist as indicated by ABG findings.		

Self-assessment	Evaluation/validation methods	Levels	Type of validation	Comments
☐Experienced ☐Need practice ☐Never done ☐Not applicable (based on scope of practice)	☐Verbal ☐Demonstration/observation ☐Practical exercise ☐Interactive class	☐Beginner ☐Intermediate ☐Expert	☐Orientation ☐Annual ☐Other _____	

_____ _____
Employee signature   Observer signature

ED—Emergency Department

Name: _____   Date: _____

Skill: Brace Application (Ice Corset)

Steps	Completed	Comments
1. Explains procedure to patient.		
2. Logrolls patient and positions corset.		
3. Inserts and flattens down ice packs.		
4. Logrolls patient to back and pulls sides of corset around to front of patient.		
5. Adjusts Velcro, wraps around abdomen.		
6. Verbalizes that ice packs changed q2 hours and prn.		
7. Stores ice packs not in use in freezer.		
8. Records name of patient and room number on ice packs.		

Self-assessment	Evaluation/validation methods	Levels	Type of validation	Comments
☐Experienced ☐Need practice ☐Never done ☐Not applicable (based on scope of practice)	☐Verbal ☐Demonstration/observation ☐Practical exercise ☐Interactive class	☐Beginner ☐Intermediate ☐Expert	☐Orientation ☐Annual ☐Other _____	

_____   _____
Employee signature   **Observer signature**

ED—EMERGENCY DEPARTMENT

Name: _____ Date: _____

Skill: Brace Application (L-S Corset)

Steps	Completed	Comments
1. Explains procedure to patient.		
2. Positions patient sitting or standing.		
3. Loosens side laces and pulls tabs.		
4. Positions brace around patient (tag at top back).		
5. Tightens up, sides laces, and pulls tabs.		
6. Adjusts for fit and patient comfort.		

Self-assessment	Evaluation/validation methods	Levels	Type of validation	Comments
☐Experienced ☐Need practice ☐Never done ☐Not applicable (based on scope of practice)	☐Verbal ☐Demonstration/observation ☐Practical exercise ☐Interactive class	☐Beginner ☐Intermediate ☐Expert	☐Orientation ☐Annual ☐Other _____	

_____ _____
Employee signature   Observer signature

COMPETENCY MANAGEMENT FOR THE EMERGENCY DEPARTMENT

ED—EMERGENCY DEPARTMENT

Name: _____   Date: _____

Skill: Brace Application (TLSO Brace)

Steps	Completed	Comments
1. Explains procedure to patient.		
2. Ensures patient is flat in bed when TLSO brace is off and when TLSO is being applied.		
3. Ensures short sleeve t-shirt is worn under TLSO.		
4. Logrolls patient to side.		
5. Positions back of TLSO brace to patient's back.		
6. Aligns waist grooves to waist and hip flare.		
7. Logrolls patient to back.		
8. Applies front of TLSO brace and aligns with back.		
9. Front slips into back on each side.		
10. Does not pinch patient's skin by pulling t-shirt taut.		
11. Fastens brace side to side with numbered Velcro fasteners.		
12. Adjusts for patient comfort.		

Self-assessment	Evaluation/validation methods	Levels	Type of validation	Comments
☐Experienced ☐Need practice ☐Never done ☐Not applicable (based on scope of practice)	☐Verbal ☐Demonstration/observation ☐Practical exercise ☐Interactive class	☐Beginner ☐Intermediate ☐Expert	☐Orientation ☐Annual ☐Other _____	

_____   _____
Employee signature   **Observer signature**

ED—EMERGENCY DEPARTMENT

Name: _____ Date: _____

Skill: Bronchoscopy Set-Up and Equipment Use

Steps	Completed	Comments
1. Scope set-up:		
a. Places sterile towel on tray		
b. Opens valves and place on tray		
c. Dons clean gloves		
d. Wipes outside of scope with alcohol soaked 4x4		
e. Places on tray and cover with sterile towel		
2. Tray set-up:		
a. NS (two bowls, one medicine cup: marked with tape)		
b. Lidocaine (one medicine cup)		
c. Xylocaine jelly		
d. Syringes (slip-tip, Kretchmer/Olbrych 2–20 cc and 2–3 cc, Fuennings's group 4–20 cc)		
e. Specitrap		
3. Additional equipment available:		
a. Forcep and histology container		
b. Brush and cytology container		
c. TBNA and 20 cc Luer-Lok and cytology container		
4. Verbalizes the need to		
a. rinse forcep in medicine cup with NS after releasing biopsy in formalin		
b. TBN, reminds physician to retract needle before removing needle from scope		
c. not submerge TBN in cytolyte to release spec		

Self-assessment	Evaluation/validation methods	Levels	Type of validation	Comments
☐Experienced ☐Need practice ☐Never done ☐Not applicable (based on scope of practice)	☐Verbal ☐Demonstration/observation ☐Practical exercise ☐Interactive class	☐Beginner ☐Intermediate ☐Expert	☐Orientation ☐Annual ☐Other _____	

_____ _____
Employee signature   Observer signature

COMPETENCY MANAGEMENT FOR THE EMERGENCY DEPARTMENT

ED—Emergency Department

Name: _____   Date: _____

Skill: | Buck's Traction |

Steps	Completed	Comments
1. Gathers equipment to add to basic frame: • Weight hanger, rope, and weight • Buck's boot by size • One 9" single-clamp bar • One 18" single-clamp bar • One pulley.		
2. Ensures patient is in good body alignment. Does not allow foot to touch end of bed.		
3. Applies Buck's boot to extremity. Bath blanket placed under leg, keeps heel free.		
4. Attaches 9" single-camp bar to basic frame upright at foot of bed extending away from patient.		
5. Attaches 18" single-clamp bar to the 9" bar to the side of the affected extremity.		
6. Attaches pulley to middle of 18" bar.		
7. Knots rope on foot plate, threads rope over pulley, and places knot for hanger. • It should be high enough so weight will not rest on floor • All knots should be taped.		
8. Removes boot by releasing Velcro straps while applying manual traction and checks skin condition (particularly heel) q8°.		
9. Places bed in William's position, modified William's position, or neutral position according to physician's preference.		
10. Documents on appropriate forms.		

Self-assessment	Evaluation/validation methods	Levels	Type of validation	Comments
☐Experienced ☐Need practice ☐Never done ☐Not applicable (based on scope of practice)	☐Verbal ☐Demonstration/observation ☐Practical exercise ☐Interactive class	☐Beginner ☐Intermediate ☐Expert	☐Orientation ☐Annual ☐Other _____	

_____   _____
Employee signature   **Observer signature**

ED—EMERGENCY DEPARTMENT

Name: _____ Date: _____

Skill: | Contrast Reaction Management |

Steps	Completed	Comments
Preinjection		
1. Describes implementation of division contrast work sheet.		
2. Lists three major patient history/physical factors considered indicators of higher potential for contrast reaction.		
3. Relates process for patient observation throughout procedure.		
Injection/procedure		
1. Lists at least three subjective patient indicators of contrast reaction.		
2. Lists at least three observable indicators of patient contrast reaction.		
3. Defines and compares mild, moderate, severe levels of contrast reaction.		
4. Categorizes the following contrast reactions according to level (mild, moderate, severe):		
a. Hives, flushing		
b. Severe hypotension		
c. Nausea, vomiting		
d. Difficulty breathing		
e. Heart stops		
f. Dysphagia/dyspnea.		
5. Sequentially describes how to appropriately manage each level of contrast reaction:		
a. Mild		
b. Moderate		
c. Severe.		

COMPETENCY MANAGEMENT FOR THE EMERGENCY DEPARTMENT

ED—Emergency Department

Communication/documentation		
1. Relates documentation processes for a contrast reaction, information, and appropriate application of each.		
a. Division contrast worksheet		
b. Contrast media reaction form		
c. Occurrence form		
d. Radiology film jacket		
e. Patient contrast reaction card.		
2. Describes oral communication process to be implemented pre and post patient contrast reaction:		
a. Radiology		
b. Referring physician		
c. Unit nursing staff		
d. Patient.		
Miscellaneous		
1. All age-specific needs were met, as applies to patient related items within this competency.		

Self-assessment	Evaluation/validation methods	Levels	Type of validation	Comments
☐Experienced ☐Need practice ☐Never done ☐Not applicable (based on scope of practice)	☐Verbal ☐Demonstration/observation ☐Practical exercise ☐Interactive class	☐Beginner ☐Intermediate ☐Expert	☐Orientation ☐Annual ☐Other _____	

_____   _____
Employee signature   **Observer signature**

ED—EMERGENCY DEPARTMENT

Name: _____ Date: _____

Skill: | Defibrillator Monitor (Heartstream XL) |

Steps	Completed	Comments
A. Defibrillation using external paddles		
1. Turns energy select knob to manual on.		
2. Applies conductive matter.		
3. Removes paddles.		
4. Applies paddles to patients chest using anterior-apex placement.		
5. Selects energy setting to 150 joules.		
6. Presses charge button on paddles.		
7. Clears area.		
8. Delivers the counter shock by simultaneously pressing the shock buttons located on the paddles until the shock is delivered.		
B. Defibrillation using multifunction defib electrode pads		
1. Turns energy select knob to manual on.		
2. Applies multifunction electrode pads to patient either anterior-apex or anterior-posterior.		
3. Connects the pads to the patient cable.		
4. Selects energy level 150 joules.		
5. Charges by pressing the charge button.		
6. Clears area.		
7. Presses shock button. Holds shock button down until shock is delivered.		
C. Sync cardioversion using external paddles		
1. Applies monitoring electrodes.		
2. Turns energy select knob to manual on.		
3. Applies conductive material.		
4. Presses sync on.		
5. Uses lead select to select the best lead that displays a large QRS complex (uses to gain control to adjust the ECG size so that the marker dot appears only with each R wave).		
6. Removes paddles and apply paddles to patient using anterior-apex placement.		

7. Selects desired energy level.		
8. Presses charge (yellow button located on apex paddle).		
9. Clears area.		
10. Delivers shock by pressing simultaneously the orange keys on both paddles. (Continues to hold down until shock is delivered. The defibrillator shocks with the next detected R wave.)		
D. Sync cardioversion using multifunction defib electrode pads		
1. Applies monitoring electrodes.		
2. Turns energy select knob to manual on.		
3. Applies multifunction defib electrode pads to the patient, either anterior-apex or anterior-posterior placement.		
4. Connects pads to the patient cable.		
5. Presses sync. on.		
6. Selects desired energy level.		
7. Presses charge.		
8. Clears area.		
9. Presses shock button. (Continues to hold down until shock is delivered. The defibrillator shocks with the next detected R wave).		
E. Pacing		
1. Applies multifunction defib electrode pads on patient using either anterior-apex or anterior-posterior placement.		
2. Connects the pads to the patient cable.		
3. Turns the energy select knob to manual on.		
4. Applies monitoring electrodes.		
5. Uses lead select to select the best lead with an easily detectable R wave.		
6. Presses pacer button (verifies that dot markers appear near the middle of the QRS complex, if not, selects another lead).		
7. Presses mode to change to fix mode or demand mode.		
8. Adjusts rate to the desired number of paced pulses per minute. (Does this by pressing up or down on the rate button to increase or decrease the number of paced pulses per minute).		

9. Presses start-stop button to start pacing.		
10. Increases the output until cardiac capture occurs (presses up arrow on the output button to increase the output in increments of 10 MA).		
11. Decreases the output to the lowest level that still maintains capture (presses down arrow on the output button to decrease the output in increments of 5 MA).		
12. Presses start-stop button to stop pacing.		
13. Presses pacer button to exit the pacing function.		
F. Miscellaneous		
1. Demonstrates how one would mark an event when administering epi, atropine, lido, other.		
2. Demonstrates how to print an event summary.		
3. Demonstrates loading printer paper.		

4. Performs a shift/system check using external paddles.
    a. Unplugs the AC cord
    b. While pressing strip button, turns the energy select knob manual on to start the test
    c. Follows the prompts on the display to proceed with the test.		

Self-assessment	Evaluation/validation methods	Levels	Type of validation	Comments
☐Experienced ☐Need practice ☐Never done ☐Not applicable (based on scope of practice)	☐Verbal ☐Demonstration/observation ☐Practical exercise ☐Interactive class	☐Beginner ☐Intermediate ☐Expert	☐Orientation ☐Annual ☐Other _____	

_____ _____
Employee signature   **Observer signature**

ED—Emergency Department

Name: _____ Date: _____

Skill: | EKG Interpretation |

Steps	Completed	Comments
1. Runs six-second strip on patient and mounts in nursing notes QS and PRN.		
2. Accurately measures and identifies normal parameters of patients rhythm strip for • rate • PR interval • QRS interval • QT interval • R-R interval • calculates QTc Documents in nurses notes q4° and prn.		
3. Identifies normal sinus rhythm.		
4. If patient is not in NSR, can identify if any of the following dysrhythmias are present (circle one if any applies): • Sinus tachycardia • Sinus bradycardia • Atrial fibrillation • Atrial flutter • Wandering atrial pacer • Premature atrial contractions • Junctional rhythm • Junctional tachycardia • Premature junctional contraction • First degree heart block • Second degree heart block Mobitz Type I • Second degree heart block Mobitz Type II • Third degree heart block (complete heart block) • Premature ventricular contraction • Ventricular tachycardia • Ventricular fibrillation • Idioventricular rhythm • Asystole.		
5. If NSR is not present, can initiate appropriate care of circled dysrhythmia according to American Heart Association's ACLS protocols.		

Self-assessment	Evaluation/validation methods	Levels	Type of validation	Comments
☐Experienced ☐Need practice ☐Never done ☐Not applicable (based on scope of practice)	☐Verbal ☐Demonstration/observation ☐Practical exercise ☐Interactive class	☐Beginner ☐Intermediate ☐Expert	☐Orientation ☐Annual ☐Other _____	

_____ _____
Employee signature   **Observer signature**

ED—EMERGENCY DEPARTMENT

Name: _____ Date: _____

Skill: | Electrocardiogram (EKG), 12-lead |

Steps	Completed	Comments
1. Identifies three interventions to safely perform an EKG.		
2. Identifies patient and describes procedure.		
3. Prepares electrode sites by briskly rubbing skin area with gauze, if necessary.		
4. Applies disposable electrodes to correct landmarks (total of 10 sites).		
5. Turns machine on and inserts disk.		
6. Assesses battery and signal integrity.		
7. Verifies appropriate settings for speed, size of EKG, and filter use.		
8. Checks supply and adds paper if needed.		
9. Identifies report type, format, and rhythm leads.		
10. Identifies correct date/time on display.		
11. Enters patient information as sequenced by machine: • "ID?" or "new patient?" _ "yes/no" • "ID?" _ addressograph plate # "name?" • "Age?" _ choose designation • "Sex?" _ choose "male/female" • "Height?" • "Weight?" • "Operator?" _ initials of operator • "Dept.?" _ unit # • "Room#?" • "Attn. Phy?" _ attending physician • "Med. Rec?" _ Bypass this screen • "Stat?" _ choose yes/no.		
12. Records on auto EKG: • Presses "auto" • Programs ID information • Stops recording with "stop" button.		
13. Records on auto EKG from the patient module: • Presses "auto" • Presses "patient module selection" • Stops recording by pressing "patient module" button.		
14. Records manual EKG: • Presses "manual" • Stops recording with either "stop" or "patient module" button.		

COMPETENCY MANAGEMENT FOR THE EMERGENCY DEPARTMENT

ED—Emergency Department

15. Copies the EKG by pressing "copy" and selecting desired analysis, if ordered.		
16. Verifies disk space availability by pressing "menu" and "check disk."		
17. Manually stores auto EKG: • Presses "menu" • Presses "store" • Formats (if appropriate).		
18. Verbalizes troubleshooting interventions for: • AC interference • Wandering baseline • Tremor/muscle artifact • Intermittent waveform • Poor print quality • Recording won't start • Dark preview screen.		
19. Describes maintenance of machine: • Cleaning procedure • Care of battery and disk.		

Self-assessment	Evaluation/validation methods	Levels	Type of validation	Comments
☐Experienced ☐Need practice ☐Never done ☐Not applicable (based on scope of practice)	☐Verbal ☐Demonstration/observation ☐Practical exercise ☐Interactive class	☐Beginner ☐Intermediate ☐Expert	☐Orientation ☐Annual ☐Other _____	

_____
Employee signature

_____
Observer signature

ED—EMERGENCY DEPARTMENT

Name: _____ Date: _____

Skill: | Foreign Body Removal |

Steps	Completed	Comments
1. Demonstrates ability to find foreign body removal equipment in department:		
a. Tripod		
b. Rat-tooth forcep		
c. Snare		
d. Basket		
e. Forcep		
f. Bezor bustor with bicap		
g. Lavage (evacuator tube).		
2. Demonstrates ability to correctly use foreign body removal equipment.		
a. Tripod		
b. Rat-tooth forcep		
c. Snare		
d. Basket		
e. Forcep		
f. Bezor bustor with bicap		
g. Lavage (evacuator tube).		

Self-assessment	Evaluation/validation methods	Levels	Type of validation	Comments
☐Experienced ☐Need practice ☐Never done ☐Not applicable (based on scope of practice)	☐Verbal ☐Demonstration/observation ☐Practical exercise ☐Interactive class	☐Beginner ☐Intermediate ☐Expert	☐Orientation ☐Annual ☐Other _____	

_____   _____
Employee signature   **Observer signature**

COMPETENCY MANAGEMENT FOR THE EMERGENCY DEPARTMENT

ED—Emergency Department

Name: _____ Date: _____

Skill: | Monitoring Lead Placement |

Steps	Completed	Comments
A. EKG monitoring		
1. Demonstrates skin preparation and application of electrodes for monitoring in Lead II, V1.		
2. Connects the EKG monitoring cable to the electrodes and to the monitor.		
3. Turns EKG monitor on.		
4. Selects the lead.		
5. Selects the waveform size.		
6. Adjusts QRS beeper volume.		
7. Selects additional options: • Filter. • Wave speed.		
8. Sets alarm limits.		
9. Turns the EKG alarms on/off.		
10. Suspends the alarms.		
11. Describes the policy for maintaining EKG alarms.		
B. Telemetry monitoring		
1. Demonstrates skin preparation and application of electrodes for monitoring in Lead II, V1.		
2. Connects the monitoring cable to the electrodes and to the telemetry pack.		
3. Turns monitor on.		
C. Arrhythmia monitoring		
1. Edits the alarms: • Validate • True/save/discard/reset • False/save/discard/reset • Store.		
D. Respirations monitoring		
1. Turns monitoring on.		
2. Adjusts size.		
3. Sets alarms.		
4. Turns alarms on/off.		
E. Admits a patient		
F. Discharges a patient		
G. Records a rhythm strip/waveform		

Self-assessment	Evaluation/validation methods	Levels	Type of validation	Comments
☐Experienced ☐Need practice ☐Never done ☐Not applicable (based on scope of practice)	☐Verbal ☐Demonstration/observation ☐Practical exercise ☐Interactive class	☐Beginner ☐Intermediate ☐Expert	☐Orientation ☐Annual ☐Other _____	

_____ _____
Employee signature   Observer signature

ED—EMERGENCY DEPARTMENT

Name: _____ Date: _____

Skill: Suture Set-Up

Steps	Completed	Comments
1. Verbalize proper wound preparation.		
2. Uses sterile technique while preparing equipment.		
3. Identifies proper solutions for disinfecting and irrigating.		
4. Explains choices of anesthetics.		
5. Describes supplies required by physicians.		
6. Role-plays patient education discharge instructions.		

Self-assessment	Evaluation/validation methods	Levels	Type of validation	Comments
☐Experienced ☐Need practice ☐Never done ☐Not applicable (based on scope of practice)	☐Verbal ☐Demonstration/observation ☐Practical exercise ☐Interactive class	☐Beginner ☐Intermediate ☐Expert	☐Orientation ☐Annual ☐Other _____	

_____ _____
Employee signature   Observer signature

COMPETENCY MANAGEMENT FOR THE EMERGENCY DEPARTMENT

ED—Emergency Department

Name: _____ Date: _____

Skill: | System 1000 Fluid Warmer (Level 1) |

Steps	Completed	Comments
1. Wears appropriate PPE.		
2. Determines unit is plugged in and grounded.		
3. Pushes the bottom of the heat exchanger into socket #1 until the bottom of the tube disappears.		
4. Pulls outside lock located by socket #2 raising socket up. Snaps heat exchanger into guide onto pole. Slides socket #2 over aluminum tube until the latch clicks.		
5. Snaps the gas filter assembly into socket #3 on side of heater assembly.		
6. Turns unit on. Verbalizes the following: • Takes three minutes for unit to be operational. • Green light indicates unit is ready. • Temperature range should be 35–38° Celsius.		
7. Verbalizes interventions for system malfunctions: • Over temperature. • Add water. • Check disposables.		
8. Introduces needle into self-sealing injection port of intravenous solution to remove air.		
9. Primes y-set, heater assembly unit, and fluid line to patient.		
10. Taps gas vent filter to release all trapped air • Verbalizes gas vent filter is to be changed every three hours while in use.		
11. Connects fluid line to patient who has a 14 G or 16 G intravenous catheter.		
12. Puts solutions under pressure • Attaches 1,000-cc bag to outside fixture of clam shell and attaches 500-cc bag (blood) to inside fixture. • Toggles switch to "on" position on top of chamber. • Verbalizes pressure will reach 300mmHg. • Toggles switch to "off" to exchange empty bag.		
13. Documents procedure and patient's response in patient care record.		

Self-assessment	Evaluation/validation methods	Levels	Type of validation	Comments
☐Experienced ☐Need practice ☐Never done ☐Not applicable (based on scope of practice)	☐Verbal ☐Demonstration/observation ☐Practical exercise ☐Interactive class	☐Beginner ☐Intermediate ☐Expert	☐Orientation ☐Annual ☐Other _____	

_____ _____
Employee signature   **Observer signature**

ED—Emergency Department

Name: _____ Date: _____

Skill: Thermacyl Fluid Warmer

Steps	Completed	Comments
1. Wears appropriate PPE.		
2. Determines unit is plugged in and grounded.		
3. Determines unit is not greater than 42 inches from the floor.		
4. Ascertains patient's fluid needs; verbalizes: • Smaller cuff delivers 350 cc/min. • Larger cuff delivers 500 cc/min.		
5. Places cuff over heating cone aligning lock-in-tab over LED window.		
6. Rotates cuff clockwise until it locks in place.		
7. Closes clamps and removes caps.		
8. Attaches male connector to female luer lock.		
9. Spikes intravenous solution and primes set.		
10. Inverts bubble trap and fills until three-quarters full.		
11. Turns upright and inserts into holder on side of unit.		
12. Attaches fluid line to patient access.		
13. Inserts remaining spike into intravenous solution or blood.		
14. Pressurizes as necessary.		
15. Turns unit on and determines functional status by series of beeps followed by silence.		
16. States set point is 40° C +/- 1° C and unit is ready in less than five minutes.		
17. Begins infusion.		
18. Documents procedure and patient's response in patient-care record.		

Self-assessment	Evaluation/validation methods	Levels	Type of validation	Comments
☐Experienced ☐Need practice ☐Never done ☐Not applicable (based on scope of practice)	☐Verbal ☐Demonstration/observation ☐Practical exercise ☐Interactive class	☐Beginner ☐Intermediate ☐Expert	☐Orientation ☐Annual ☐Other _____	

_____   _____
Employee signature   **Observer signature**

COMPETENCY MANAGEMENT FOR THE EMERGENCY DEPARTMENT

ED—Emergency Department

Name: _____   Date: _____

Skill: Thrombolytic Therapy

Steps	Completed	Comments
Before therapy has begun:		
1. Establishes two vascular access sites (one may be HL) and checks sites at least q 15 min.		
2. Verbalizes contraindications (uncontrolled hypertension, history of bleeding ulcer, active internal bleeding, recent intracranial/intraspinal surgery or trauma, intracranial neoplasm, AV malformation, aneurysm).		
3. Uses caution/gentleness when moving patient.		
4. Obtains baseline VS and neuro status.		
5. Obtains baseline laboratory values (Hemogram, PT, PTT, fibrinogen, electrolytes, CPK).		
6. Avoids repeated needle punctures (blood draws are grouped, avoid IM injections if possible).		
During therapy infusion:		
1. Monitors VS and neuro status q 15 min and notifies physician of change immediately.		
2. Checks arm under blood pressure cuff for ecchymosis q 1 hour. Rotates cuff prn.		
3. Monitor for signs of reperfusion (decreased chest pain, resolution of ST elevation, development of arrhythmias).		
4. Looks for subtle signs of bleeding (tachycardia, orthostatic hypotension).		
5. Assesses all body drainage for presence of blood and record findings (urine/stool/emesis/gastric drainage).		
6. Monitors lab values (H&H, PT, PTT, other coag, BUN, Creat, CPK).		
7. Applies pressure to all venipuncture sites for at least five minutes.		
8. Identifies risk factors for clot information (elderly, diabetic, smoking hx., elevated lipids, hypertension, sedentary lifestyle).		
After therapy is completed:		
1. Monitors VS and neuro check's q 15 min x 2 hr then q 1 hr x 2 then q 2 hr. x 24 hrs.		
2. Monitors lab values using second IV site q 12 h x 24 h the qd x 2.		
3. Assesses for subtle signs of bleeding (as above) q 12h.		
4. Assesses for signs of reocclusion and notifies physician immediately (recurrent chest pain, ST segment elevation, diaphoresis, nausea, arrhythmia).		
5. Educates the patient about the current therapy and also the probable use of a "blood thinner" at home.		

Self-assessment	Evaluation/validation methods	Levels	Type of validation	Comments
☐Experienced ☐Need practice ☐Never done ☐Not applicable (based on scope of practice)	☐Verbal ☐Demonstration/observation ☐Practical exercise ☐Interactive class	☐Beginner ☐Intermediate ☐Expert	☐Orientation ☐Annual ☐Other _____	

_____   _____
Employee signature   Observer signature

ED—EMERGENCY DEPARTMENT

Name: _____ Date: _____

Skill: Tourniquet Safety

Steps	Completed	Comments
1. Checks pressure in tanks (tank changed if below 1,000psi).		
2. Checks pressure gauge for accuracy.		
3. Sets pressure gauge for procedure.		
4. Per surgeon's preference, properly applies padding to leg/arm.		
5. Applies proper size of tourniquet cuff.		
6. Inflates cuff for procedure and checks pressure gauge for accuracy.		
7. When applicable, notifies surgeon when tourniquet has been in place for one hour (every 30 minutes thereafter).		
8. Following procedure, turns off tourniquet gauge and removes cuff.		
9. Turns tank valve down and off.		
10. Completes appropriate documentation for tourniquet use and disconnects (skin condition pre and post noted and documented).		

Self-assessment	Evaluation/validation methods	Levels	Type of validation	Comments
☐Experienced ☐Need practice ☐Never done ☐Not applicable (based on scope of practice)	☐Verbal ☐Demonstration/observation ☐Practical exercise ☐Interactive class	☐Beginner ☐Intermediate ☐Expert	☐Orientation ☐Annual ☐Other _____	

_____ _____
Employee signature   **Observer signature**

COMPETENCY MANAGEMENT FOR THE EMERGENCY DEPARTMENT

ED—Emergency Department

Name: _____ Date: _____

Skill: | Triage — Diarrhea |

Steps	Completed	Comments
1. Determines the following information: • Duration of diarrhea • Frequency of stool • Consistency of stool.		
2. Questions patient about presence of: • Abdominal pain • Nausea/vomiting.		
3. Determines if a temperature elevation exists.		
4. Lists medications patient is currently taking.		
5. Ascertains CD4 count.		
6. Documents findings accurately.		
7. Determines if any travel time (out of state or overseas).		
8. Determines if any other household members with diarrhea.		

Self-assessment	Evaluation/validation methods	Levels	Type of validation	Comments
☐ Experienced ☐ Need practice ☐ Never done ☐ Not applicable (based on scope of practice)	☐ Verbal ☐ Demonstration/observation ☐ Practical exercise ☐ Interactive class	☐ Beginner ☐ Intermediate ☐ Expert	☐ Orientation ☐ Annual ☐ Other _____	

Employee signature _____ Observer signature _____

ED—EMERGENCY DEPARTMENT

Name: _____ Date: _____

Skill: | Triage — Upper Respiratory Infection |

Steps	Completed	Comments
1. Determines if a temperature elevation exists.		
2. Identifies presence of productive cough.		
3. Questions patient if shortness of breath exists.		
4. Determines start of symptoms.		
5. Lists medications patient is currently taking.		
6. Ascertains CD4 count.		
7. Documents findings accurately.		

Self-assessment	Evaluation/validation methods	Levels	Type of validation	Comments
☐Experienced ☐Need practice ☐Never done ☐Not applicable (based on scope of practice)	☐Verbal ☐Demonstration/observation ☐Practical exercise ☐Interactive class	☐Beginner ☐Intermediate ☐Expert	☐Orientation ☐Annual ☐Other _____	

_____ _____
Employee signature   Observer signature

ED—Emergency Department

Name: _____   Date: _____

Skill: **Welch Allyn Ear Wash System**

Steps	Completed	Comments
Set-up		
1. Unscrews current aerator and its washer from the faucet.		
2. Attaches the snap aerator.		
3. Matches the colors and connects the tubing to the chamber.		
4. Sets the temperature to 90–100 degrees Fahrenheit.		
5. Depresses the actuator on the handle and observes the sensor change color from blue to white.		
Use		
1. Attaches an ear tip to the interface on the irrigation handle with the tab side up.		
2. Inserts the ear tip into the entrance of the ear canal.		
3. Irrigates the canal by aiming stream of water toward ear canal walls by rotating the handle around the ear canal.		
4. Checks patient for comfort level.		
5. Maintains temperature of the irrigating water.		
6. Releases actuator and keeps the ear tip by the ear canal for five to 10 seconds to vacuum residual water.		
Cleaning		
1. Prepares a four-cup solution of soap and water.		
2. Detaches the chamber from the faucet. Pours half of the solution into the chamber.		
3. Replaces the chamber on the faucet head and submerges the handle where the tip attaches into the remainder of the solution.		
4. Turns on the water. Squeezes the actuator to allow the solution to flow from the handle into the container. The		

suction line removes the solution. Continues this process for five minutes.		
5. Turns the water off and removes both tubes from the chamber.		
6. Disconnects the hoses from the chamber. Holding the handle higher than the tube and squeezing the actuator will allow the water to run out of the open end into the sink.		
7. Removes the chamber from the faucet. Allows the chamber to drip dry. Replaces the unit in its holding container.		
Disassembly		
1. Turns off the faucet and disconnect tubing.		
2. Detaches the unit from the faucet.		
3. Holds the handle higher than the tubing and squeezed the actuator to remove remaining water.		

Self-assessment	Evaluation/validation methods	Levels	Type of validation	Comments
☐Experienced ☐Need practice ☐Never done ☐Not applicable (based on scope of practice)	☐Verbal ☐Demonstration/observation ☐Practical exercise ☐Interactive class	☐Beginner ☐Intermediate ☐Expert	☐Orientation ☐Annual ☐Other _____	

_____   _____
Employee signature   **Observer signature**

ED—Emergency Department

Name: _____ Date: _____

Skill: | Women's Health Infant Safety/Abduction/Code Pink |

Steps	Completed	Comments
I. Prevention		
A. All accesses secured with alarm locks.		
B. Camera in stairwells.		
C. Personnel wear ID tags.		
D. Infant wears ID bracelets.		
E. Photos taken of newborn.		
F. Footprints taken of newborn.		
G. Drills for Code Pink.		
II. Code Pink drill		
A. Call 53277 (protective services).		
B. Code Pink announced over call system and other units.		
C. Infant head count initiated.		
D. 7p–7a shift		
1. Check location of infants.		
2. Record on checklist.		
3. Notify security of count.		
E. 7a–7p shift		
1. Return babies to nursery.		
2. Initiate head count.		
3. Notify security of count.		
III. Actual abduction		
A. Calls protective services of suspicious behavior.		
B. Alerts protective services of abduction occurring.		
C. Announces "Code Pink."		
D. Asks if witnessed.		

Self-assessment	Evaluation/validation methods	Levels	Type of validation	Comments
☐Experienced ☐Need practice ☐Never done ☐Not applicable (based on scope of practice)	☐Verbal ☐Demonstration/observation ☐Practical exercise ☐Interactive class	☐Beginner ☐Intermediate ☐Expert	☐Orientation ☐Annual ☐Other _____	

_____ _____
Employee signature   Observer signature

ALL (General, All Units)

Contents

1. Accurate Pressure Measurements 145
2. Age-Specific Competency Checklist RN-LPN 146
3. Age-Specific Competency Checklist SA-AA 148
4. Annual Competency Performance—Cleaning Delivery Rooms 150
5. Annual Competency Performance—Quality of Instruction 151
6. Blood Glucose Meter 152
7. Blood Pressure Measurement 154
8. Code Management/Med-Surg 155
9. Emergency Preparedness 157
10. Hand Washing 158
11. Oximeter (Whole Blood O_2 Saturation) 159
12. Oxygen Administration 161
13. Telephone Skills 162
14. Telephone Skills (Problem Solving) 163
15. Use Automated External Defibrillator (Heartstream FR2) 164

ALL—GENERAL, ALL UNITS

Name: _____   Date: _____

Skill: | Accurate Pressure Measurements |

Steps	Completed	Comments
1. Both transducers are mounted together on manifold/pole or on table rail (depending on room).		
2. Measures/locates midaxillary line.		
3. Transfers midaxillary line measurement to thigh…if not at top of thigh, marks drape with sterile marker to indicate midaxillary level.		
4. Opens both stopcocks to air at the mark on drape to zero pressures.		
5. Records table height at this point and records all pressures at this table height (only until injector is mounted on table).		
6. Calibrates both to 100 at Cathcor by pushing button on Medex back plate (may not need for every case).		
7. Returns table to zeroing height during pressure measurement (only until injector mounted on table can also re-zero with stopcocks). Before doing a simultaneous pressure measurement, re-zoning is recommended, using top of thigh or drape mark as a reference.		
8. Reminds physician to hold stopcock at the same location so zero is correct during pressure measurement.		

Self-assessment	Evaluation/validation methods	Levels	Type of validation	Comments
☐Experienced ☐Need practice ☐Never done ☐Not applicable (based on scope of practice)	☐Verbal ☐Demonstration/observation ☐Practical exercise ☐Interactive class	☐Beginner ☐Intermediate ☐Expert	☐Orientation ☐Annual ☐Other _____	

_____   _____
Employee signature   Observer signature

COMPETENCY MANAGEMENT FOR THE EMERGENCY DEPARTMENT

ALL—GENERAL, ALL UNITS

Name: _____ Date: _____

Skill: | Age-Specific Competency Checklist RN/LPN |

Steps	Completed	Comments
1. Alters care given on age-specific needs.		
A. Physical		
Adolescent – increases need for nourishment/nutrition.		
Early adulthood – alters diet, decreases amount of food.		
Middle adult – provides assistance with ambulation, provides moisture, keeps temperature set for comfort.		
Late adult – close observation of vital signs, I&O stays alert for drug-drug interactions.		
B. Motor/sensory adaptation		
Adolescent – assists with ambulation, provides for sleep.		
Early adulthood – ensures decreased background noise, encourages use of glasses.		
Middle adult – speaks loudly, assists with ambulation.		
Late adult – does not rush patient; provides glasses, hearing aids for assistance.		
C. Cognitive		
Adolescent – speaks to patient as an adult not a child.		
Early adulthood – identifies learning preferences.		
Middle adult – alters patient education techniques.		

Late adult — encourages participation in society, social groups.		
D. Psychosocial		
Adolescence — encourages peers to visit/phone, explores feelings with patients.		
Early adulthood — explores how illness will stress job, family, and responsibilities.		
Middle adult — helps patient identify stressors and his or her relationship to illness		
Late adult — assesses patient's place in society, addresses concerns.		

Self-assessment	Evaluation/validation methods	Levels	Type of validation	Comments
☐Experienced ☐Need practice ☐Never done ☐Not applicable (based on scope of practice)	☐Verbal ☐Demonstration/observation ☐Practical exercise ☐Interactive class	☐Beginner ☐Intermediate ☐Expert	☐Orientation ☐Annual ☐Other _____	

_____ _____
Employee signature   **Observer signature**

ALL—GENERAL, ALL UNITS

Name: _____   Date: _____

Skill: | Age-Specific Competency Checklist SA/AA |

Steps	Completed	Comments
1. Alters care based on age-specific needs.		
A. Physical		
Adolescent – provides snacks		
Early adulthood – provides alternative foods within diet.		
Middle adult – sets room temperature for patient comfort.		
Late adult – measures urine output, reports changes to nurse.		
B. Motor/sensory adaptation		
Adolescent – assists with ambulation, provides for rest.		
Early adulthood – keeps area quiet.		
Middle adult – speaks slowly, assists with ambulation.		
Late adult – does not rush patient.		
C. Cognitive		
Adolescent – treats patient as an adult.		
Early adulthood – helps patient to alleviate boredom.		
Middle adult – repeats instructions as needed—answers questions.		
Late adult – encourages activities.		

D. Psychosocial		
Adolescent – encourages patient to talk, participate.		
Early adulthood – participates in identification of stress of patient and reports to nurse.		
Middle adult – participates in identification of stressors and reports to nurse.		
Late adult – encourages participant in ADLs—offers to help when needed.		

Self-assessment	Evaluation/validation methods	Levels	Type of validation	Comments
☐Experienced ☐Need practice ☐Never done ☐Not applicable (based on scope of practice)	☐Verbal ☐Demonstration/observation ☐Practical exercise ☐Interactive class	☐Beginner ☐Intermediate ☐Expert	☐Orientation ☐Annual ☐Other _____	

_____   _____
Employee signature   **Observer signature**

ALL—GENERAL, ALL UNITS

Name: _____ Date: _____

Skill: **Annual Competency Performance—Cleaning Delivery Rooms**

Steps	Completed	Comments
Always use body fluid isolation precautions!		
1. Obtains housekeeping cart and bring to room.		
2. Collects contaminated delivery instruments and takes to dirty utility room.		
3. Collects all soiled linens and places in linen bag.		
a. Linen bags should be lined with a clear plastic bag for the protection of the laundry personnel.		
4. Collects all white bag trash.		
a. Knots bag twice to prevent contents from spilling.		
5. Collects all red bag trash (biohazard trash).		
a. Soiled drapes and paper from the immediate delivery area.		
b. Soiled drapes, suction tubing, O_2 mask, bulb suction from the infant warmer.		
c. Red bag trash from bathroom.		
6. Uses a disinfectant-soaked blue towel for each separate piece of furniture:		
a. Infant warmer.		
b. Patient bed — removes foot mattress and wipe down stirrups. Makes sure to examine all surfaces for spillage, including wheels and frame.		
c. Delivery table.		
d. Bedside stand.		
e. Overbed table.		
f. Telephone.		
7. Mops floor thoroughly with disinfectant solution, including bathroom.		
8. Wipes down bathroom sink/commode with Aspetizyme.		
9. After all disinfected surfaces are dry:		
a. Replaces all white and red trash bags.		
b. Makes bed with fresh linen.		
c. Places fresh patient gown and clothing bag on the made bed.		
d. Replaces any suction tubing/suction canisters (infant or adult).		
e. Restocks room as necessary (including blankets/pillows).		
f. Performs final room check (bed in low position and room prepped and presentable).		
g. This checklist will be monitored twice annually.		

Self-assessment	Evaluation/validation methods	Levels	Type of validation	Comments
☐ Experienced ☐ Need practice ☐ Never done ☐ Not applicable (based on scope of practice)	☐ Verbal ☐ Demonstration/observation ☐ Practical exercise ☐ Interactive class	☐ Beginner ☐ Intermediate ☐ Expert	☐ Orientation ☐ Annual ☐ Other _____	

_____   _____
Employee signature   **Observer signature**

ALL—GENERAL, ALL UNITS

Name: _____ **Date:** _____

Skill: Annual Competency Performance—Quality of Instruction

Steps	Completed	Comments
1. Completes documentation within appropriate time frame.		
2. Maintains records that are		
a. accurate.		
b. complete.		
c. concise.		
d. objective.		
e. legible.		
3. Documents participant reaction to presentation.		

Self-assessment	Evaluation/validation methods	Levels	Type of validation	Comments
☐Experienced ☐Need practice ☐Never done ☐Not applicable (based on scope of practice)	☐Verbal ☐Demonstration/observation ☐Practical exercise ☐Interactive class	☐Beginner ☐Intermediate ☐Expert	☐Orientation ☐Annual ☐Other _____	

_____ _____
Employee signature **Observer signature**

COMPETENCY MANAGEMENT FOR THE EMERGENCY DEPARTMENT

ALL—GENERAL, ALL UNITS

Name: _____ Date: _____

Skill: | Blood Glucose Meter |

Steps	Completed	Comments
Quality control		
1. Demonstrates how to properly clean meter.		
2. Turns on meter and correctly verifies test strip code.		
3. Performs check strip validation correctly.		
4. Performs high & low controls according to instructions/prompts.		
5. Explains or demonstrates how to appropriately document quality control (QC) results (QC log).		
6. Explains or demonstrates how to correct a "failed" QC result.		
7. Explains/demonstrates how to document the corrective action on a "failed" QC result.		
Patient testing		
1. Properly identifies patient.		
2. Describes procedure to patient.		
3. Wears appropriate personal protective equipment (PPE) when collecting/handling sample.		
4. Assesses patient's fingertips and chooses appropriate site for sample collection.		
5. Explains or demonstrates purpose of test code chip and how to replace.		
6. Turns on meter and verifies test strip code correctly.		
7. Correctly inserts test strip into meter.		
8. Correctly obtains blood sample from fingerstick.		
9. Applies sufficient amount of blood sample to test strip.		
10. Documents patient result on appropriate form/chart.		
11. Provides appropriate postfingerstick care to patient.		

12. Discards testing materials in appropriate containers (i.e., lancet, test strip, etc.).		
13. States critical value ranges when a sample is to be collected and sent to the laboratory for analysis.		
14. Explains or demonstrates the collection of a confirmation sample.		
15. Reviewed current procedure for relevant revisions.		

Self-assessment	Evaluation/validation methods	Levels	Type of validation	Comments
☐Experienced ☐Need practice ☐Never done ☐Not applicable (based on scope of practice)	☐Verbal ☐Demonstration/observation ☐Practical exercise ☐Interactive class	☐Beginner ☐Intermediate ☐Expert	☐Orientation ☐Annual ☐Other _____	

_____   _____
Employee signature   **Observer signature**

ALL—GENERAL, ALL UNITS

Name: _____   Date: _____

Skill: | Blood Pressure Measurement |

Steps	Completed	Comments
1. Identifies patient and explains procedure.		
2. Selects an appropriately sized blood-pressure cuff for the patient.		
3. Locates the brachial artery (inner aspect of the elbow).		
4. Places cuff so the inflatable bag is centered over the brachial artery and the lower edge of the cuff is about one to two inches above site.		
5. Wraps cuff around the arm snugly; fastens it securely or tucks the end of the cuff well under the preceding wrapping.		
6. Places the stethoscope into ears and closes the screw valve on the air pump.		
7. With the fingertips of left hand, feels for the pulse over brachial artery. Places stethoscope firmly but with little pressure over area.		
8. Palpates brachial artery with left hand and pumps bulb until gauge rises about 30 mmHg above the point at which the brachial pulse disappears, or pumps bulb until gauge is 30 mmHg above the point that the BP has been running.		
9. Uses the valve on the bulb to release air slowly, and notes the point on the manometer at which the first of two consecutive beats is heard (systolic pressure).		
10. Continues to release air in the cuff evenly and slowly. Notes the reading on the manometer when all sounds disappear (diastolic pressure).		
11. Allows the remaining air to escape quickly and removes the cuff.		
12. Documents blood pressure reading on graphic record.		

Self-assessment	Evaluation/validation methods	Levels	Type of validation	Comments
☐Experienced ☐Need practice ☐Never done ☐Not applicable (based on scope of practice)	☐Verbal ☐Demonstration/observation ☐Practical exercise ☐Interactive class	☐Beginner ☐Intermediate ☐Expert	☐Orientation ☐Annual ☐Other _____	

_____   _____
Employee signature   **Observer signature**

ALL—GENERAL, ALL UNITS

Name: _____ Date: _____

Skill: | Code Management/Med-Surg. |

Steps	Completed	Comments
1. Assesses unresponsiveness. • Checks for breathing.		
2. If patient is breathing: • Applies O_2 via NC. • Places heart monitor on patient. • Places pulse oximeter on patient. • Informs physician of episode.		
3. Checks for pulse: • No pulse		
4. Calls for help and AED if applicable: • Help should bring code cart.		
5. Initiative code: picks up in house phone and calls the "team" or delegates to another staff member.		
6. Verbalizes correct phone number to call.		
7. Utilizes ABCs of CPR. • One rescuer: Begins to use the Ambu bag on patient & one-person CPR. • Two rescuers: Places back board under patient & begins two-person CPR. • Three rescuers: Places heart monitor on patient. Sets up suction set ups and gets intubation equipment ready to go. Starts peripheral IV of N/S if not already started.		
8. RN assumes leadership role giving directions to staff: • Gets patient's chart to bedside. • Is ready with short summary of patient status for "team members." • Documents activities performed during team on Team/Surgical Record.		
9. "Team" members: • Identifies rhythm, assesses pulse.		
10. Delivers pre-cardial thump, if appropriate.		
11. Defibrillates according to ACLS protocols. • Turns defibrillator on. • Charges to appropriate setting. • Places paddles. • Clears area. • Delivers countershock. • Assesses patient.		

ALL—GENERAL, ALL UNITS

12. Directs "team" members (if not already done) to: • Perform compressions. • Initiate IV. • Insert and secure endotracheal tube. • Verify correct tube placement. • Document team event.		
13. Initiates appropriate drug therapy • CPA — Asystole. • CPA — V-fib/pulseless V tach.		
14. Cardioverts as indicated: • Turns on synchronizer. • Observes synchronization maker. • Charges cardioverter to appropriate setting. • Places paddles. • Clears area. • Delivers countershock. • Assesses patient		
15. Applies transcutaneous pacing at a rate of 70 ppm: • Attaches pacing electrodes to patient and pacemaker cable. • Attaches EKG leads from pacemaker. • Turns unit on. • Notes pace "sensing," adjusts if appropriate. • Selects rate. • Selects output. • Starts pacing; evaluates capture. • To defibrillate, stops pacing.		
16. When rhythm and pulse restored, follow up on: • Stability of rhythm. • Pulse, blood pressure. • Status of respirations. • Transport as appropriate. • IVs and medications infusing. • Ventilator settings. • Post arrest orders and care.		
17. Verifies documentation utilizing team record.		

Self-assessment	Evaluation/validation methods	Levels	Type of validation	Comments
☐Experienced ☐Need practice ☐Never done ☐Not applicable (based on scope of practice)	☐Verbal ☐Demonstration/observation ☐Practical exercise ☐Interactive class	☐Beginner ☐Intermediate ☐Expert	☐Orientation ☐Annual ☐Other _____	

_____   _____
Employee signature   **Observer signature**

ALL—GENERAL, ALL UNITS

Name: _____   Date: _____

Skill: | Emergency Preparedness |

Steps	Completed	Comments
1. Assesses if a medical emergency exists: physical assessment (patient responsiveness, LOC, vitals); historical assessment (diabetes, autonomic neuropathy, hypotensive episodes).		
2. Identifies correct pathway cardiac rehab emergency treatment algorithm.		
3. Demonstrates ventilation technique via Resusci mask.		
4. Demonstrates O_2 to ambu bag and nasal cannula hook-up.		
5. Demonstrates fitting patient with nasal cannula.		
6. Performs BLS ABCs and one cycle of rescue breathing and cardiac compressions.		
7. Identifies team code number to call.		
8. Demonstrates technique for transferring patient from telemetry to defibrillator leads, selects limb and augmented lead positions, runs an ECG strip.		
9. Transports team cart and gurney from exam room to exercise area.		
10. Identifies team cart components: emergency drug box, phase IV solutions, IV start sets, pulse oximeter.		
11. Demonstrates: placement of conductive defib pads on the chest wall, placement and pressure on the defib paddles, and the correct sequence of ACLS defibrillation shocks.		
12. Demonstrates technique for transferring patient to gurney and transporting patient to exam room or ED department.		

Self-assessment	Evaluation/validation methods	Levels	Type of validation	Comments
☐Experienced ☐Need practice ☐Never done ☐Not applicable (based on scope of practice)	☐Verbal ☐Demonstration/observation ☐Practical exercise ☐Interactive class	☐Beginner ☐Intermediate ☐Expert	☐Orientation ☐Annual ☐Other _____	

_____   _____
Employee signature   **Observer signature**

COMPETENCY MANAGEMENT FOR THE EMERGENCY DEPARTMENT

ALL—GENERAL, ALL UNITS

Name: _____ Date: _____

Skill: | Hand Washing |

Steps	Completed	Comments
1. Checks that sink area is supplied with soap and paper towels.		
2. Exposes wrist area, rolls up sleeves and slides watch up arm.		
3. Stands a few inches away from sink.		
4. Turns on faucet and regulates water temperature.		
5. Wets hands and applies recommended amount of soap or detergent.		
6. Washes hands and wrists thoroughly for 10–15 seconds, keeping fingertips pointed down and cleaning under fingernails if necessary.		
7. Rinses hands and wrists thoroughly, keeping fingertips pointed down.		
8. Dries hands and wrists thoroughly with paper towel.		
9. Discards paper towel in wastebasket.		
10. Uses another paper towel to turn off faucets.		
11. Discards paper towel in wastebasket.		

Self-assessment	Evaluation/validation methods	Levels	Type of validation	Comments
☐Experienced ☐Need practice ☐Never done ☐Not applicable (based on scope of practice)	☐Verbal ☐Demonstration/observation ☐Practical exercise ☐Interactive class	☐Beginner ☐Intermediate ☐Expert	☐Orientation ☐Annual ☐Other _____	

Employee signature _____ Observer signature _____

ALL—GENERAL, ALL UNITS

Name: _____ Date: _____

Skill: Oximeter (Whole Blood O₂ Saturation)

Steps	Completed	Comments
1. States when to perform electronic quality control (QC) testing (every 24 hrs of patient testing).		
2. Checks that instrument switch is in O₂ saturation position.		
3. Allows machine to warm up for appropriate time (approx. 15 minutes).		
4. Correctly inserts appropriate QC filter wand (QC1) when "INS" is displayed.		
5. Demonstrates how to perform QC2 & QC3 (remove filter, press green start button, and wait for INS to be displayed).		
6. Demonstrates how and where to appropriately document QC filter results.		
7. States or demonstrates what to do when "RMV" appears on display.		
8. States or demonstrates what to do when "ERE" appears on display (results are "out of range").		
9. States or demonstrates what to do when QC is out of range.		
Patient testing		
10. Wears appropriate personal protective equipment when collecting and handling specimen.		
11. Demonstrates principles of aseptic technique when collecting specimen.		
12. States when instrument is ready to perform patient testing ("RDY" is displayed).		
13. Prepares cuvette by attaching filter.		

ALL—GENERAL, ALL UNITS

14. Obtains the appropriate amount of specimen (1 cc & no air bubbles)		
15. Correctly attaches syringe to cuvette (nonfiltered end) and depresses plunger to fill cuvette.		
16. Presses START button on oximeter.		
17. Inserts cuvette (with syringe) when "INS" is displayed.		
18. States and demonstrates how to handle patient results (verbally to cardiologist, record on patient log and nursing record).		
19. Performs appropriate patient post care.		
20. Disposes of equipment in appropriate biohazard container.		
21. States how to collect patient sample from central line (withdraw and discard).		
22. States what to do when result does not correlate with patient therapy.		

Self-assessment	Evaluation/validation methods	Levels	Type of validation	Comments
☐Experienced ☐Need practice ☐Never done ☐Not applicable (based on scope of practice)	☐Verbal ☐Demonstration/observation ☐Practical exercise ☐Interactive class	☐Beginner ☐Intermediate ☐Expert	☐Orientation ☐Annual ☐Other _____	

_____   _____
Employee signature   **Observer signature**

ALL—GENERAL, ALL UNITS

OK

Name: _____ **Date:** _____

Skill: | Oxygen Administration |

Steps	Completed	Comments
1. Verifies the physician's order.		
2. Washes hands.		
3. Obtains the required equipment:		
a. Oxygen flowmeter		
b. Humidifier (over 4 liters)		
c. Sterile water (over 4 liters)		
d. Oxygen connecting tubing (if needed)		
e. Oxygen administration device		
f. No Smoking sign(s)		
4. Identifies the patient and explains procedure.		
5. Adjusts the device to the ordered level.		
6. Applies the device to the patient.		
7. Confirms F_iO_2 as appropriate.		
8. Leaves the patient area clean and safe after disposing of excess equipment.		
9. Washes hands before leaving room.		
10. Documents equipment, concentration, or liter flow in the patient's chart.		

Self-assessment	Evaluation/validation methods	Levels	Type of validation	Comments
☐Experienced ☐Need practice ☐Never done ☐Not applicable (based on scope of practice)	☐Verbal ☐Demonstration/observation ☐Practical exercise ☐Interactive class	☐Beginner ☐Intermediate ☐Expert	☐Orientation ☐Annual ☐Other _____	

_____ _____
Employee signature **Observer signature**

COMPETENCY MANAGEMENT FOR THE EMERGENCY DEPARTMENT

ALL—GENERAL, ALL UNITS

Name: _____ Date: _____

Skill: | Telephone Skills |

Steps	Completed	Comments
1. Answers the telephone in three rings or less.		
2. Identifies self by department, title, and name in appropriate professional business tone and language.		
3. Asks caller how one can be of service (example: "How may I help you today?").		
4. Demonstrates placing caller on hold, checking back every 30 seconds or less while looking for additional information for the caller.		
5. Demonstrates transferring a call when the caller has accessed one's department incorrectly.		
6. Demonstrates taking a message: records caller's name, nature of message, telephone number, etc.		
7. Closes conversation with offers of any other assistance and thank you.		

Self-assessment	Evaluation/validation methods	Levels	Type of validation	Comments
☐Experienced ☐Need practice ☐Never done ☐Not applicable (based on scope of practice)	☐Verbal ☐Demonstration/observation ☐Practical exercise ☐Interactive class	☐Beginner ☐Intermediate ☐Expert	☐Orientation ☐Annual ☐Other _____	

_____   _____
Employee signature   **Observer signature**

ALL—GENERAL, ALL UNITS

ok

Name: _____ Date: _____

Skill: | Telephone Skills (Problem Solving)

Steps	Completed	Comments
1. Answers routine telephone calls by the third ring in a friendly manner by identifying his or her name and department.		
2. Refers to interdepartmental phone book and class schedules to help locate any employees or meetings in our buildings. Asks for clarification.		
3. Utilizes other staff members for telephone coverage while away from the desk area/has someone sit at the reception desk to cover the phone calls.		
4. Before leaving for lunch or break, asks who is available to cover the phone. Gives a time reference as to when he or she is leaving and will be returning.		
5. Notifies person when he or she returns.		
6. Keeps Rolodex up-to-date.		
7. Retrieves voicemail message in a timely manner and responds/follows through accordingly.		

Self-assessment	Evaluation/validation methods	Levels	Type of validation	Comments
☐ Experienced ☐ Need practice ☐ Never done ☐ Not applicable (based on scope of practice)	☐ Verbal ☐ Demonstration/observation ☐ Practical exercise ☐ Interactive class	☐ Beginner ☐ Intermediate ☐ Expert	☐ Orientation ☐ Annual ☐ Other _____	

_____ _____
Employee signature   **Observer signature**

COMPETENCY MANAGEMENT FOR THE EMERGENCY DEPARTMENT

ALL—GENERAL, ALL UNITS

Name: _____ Date: _____

Skill: | Use of Automated External Defibrillator (Heartstream FR2) |

Steps	Completed	Comments
1. Assesses the patient for unconsciousness, no breathing, and no detectable pulse.		
2. Turns on the Heartstream FR2.		
3. Simulates proper skin prep prior to pads placement.		
4. Correctly places defibrillation pads.		
5. Plugs the pads connector into Heartstream FR2's connector port.		
6. Ensures no one touches the patient when Heartstream FR2 is analyzing.		
7. Verbally and visually clears the patient prior to delivering shock.		
8. Presses shock button when advised.		
9. Assesses patient for presence of a pulse when the Heartstream FR2 gives a "No Shock Advised" message.		

Self-assessment	Evaluation/validation methods	Levels	Type of validation	Comments
☐Experienced ☐Need practice ☐Never done ☐Not applicable (based on scope of practice)	☐Verbal ☐Demonstration/observation ☐Practical exercise ☐Interactive class	☐Beginner ☐Intermediate ☐Expert	☐Orientation ☐Annual ☐Other _____	

_____ _____
Employee signature   **Observer signature**